D. E. S.

Also by Robert Meyers

Like Normal People

D. E. S.
The Bitter Pill

Robert Meyers

Seaview/Putnam
New York

Library of Congress Cataloging in Publication Data

Meyers, Robert.
    D. E. S., the bitter pill.

    Bibliography: p.
    Includes index.
    1. Diethylstilbestrol—Toxicology. 2. Diethylstilbestrol—Side effects.
3. Fetus—Effect of drugs on. 4. Vagina—Cancer. 5. Generative organs—Abnormalities. I. Title. II. Title: D.E.S., the bitter pill.
RA1242.D48M49 1983   363.1′94   83-377
ISBN 0-399-31008-8

Printed in the United States of America

ACKNOWLEDGMENTS

This lengthy and complex project would not have been possible without the help of dozens of patient people all over the United States as well as in the United Kingdom. Chief among these are the many people with an intimate and personal knowledge of DES: the women who took it during their pregnancies, and the women and men born to them. It is their stories, told in full, that may serve to bring the impact of the DES experience to the awareness of others. All of the names used in this book are the real names of real people. For their courage in telling me their stories, and their help in making sure I had recorded everything accurately, I am deeply grateful.

From the very beginning of this project I was aided by the two nationwide consumer organizations DES Action and the DES Registry. At DES Action I wish to thank Nancy Adess, Pat Cody, and Dolores Wallgren. At the DES Registry I wish to thank Phyllis Wetherill. Dolores Wallgren and Phyllis Wetherill were both enormously generous in taking time from their busy schedules to assist me in my research, respond to my telephone calls, and track down bits and pieces of information I needed. Their contributions cannot be minimized. During one research trip to California, Laura Minor, in Los Angeles, set up interviews for me with DES-exposed people in their areas and helped me organize my time efficiently.

Within the field of medicine and research I would like to thank each of the individuals mentioned in the text for taking time to speak with me, either in person or over the phone, helping me understand the impact of their work, and then helping me translate that information into a readily understandable vocabulary without losing any precision of thought.

I would like to thank especially Howard Ulfelder, M.D., Joe V. Meigs Professor of Gynecology at Harvard Medical School; Ann Brace Barnes, M.D., Massachusetts General Hospital; Arthur L. Herbst, M.D., chairman of the Department of Gynecology, University of Chicago School of Medicine; Duane E. Townsend, M.D., associate director, Gynecologic Oncology, Cedars-Sinai Medical Center, Los Angeles; William G. Karow, M.D., Southern California Fertility Clinic, Los Angeles; George Speck, M.D., Alexandria, Virginia; George Van Siclen Smith, M.D., and Olive Watkins Smith, Ph.D., Boston, Massachusetts; Karl John Karnaky, M.D., The Obstetrical and Gynecological Research Foundation and Research Institute, Houston, Texas; Harry C. Miller, M.D., chairman of the Department of Urology, George Washington University, Washington, D.C.; Bruce Stadel, M.D., National Institute of Child Health and Human Development; Sidney M. Wolfe, M.D., head of Public Citizen's Health Research Group; and Stanley J. Robboy, M.D., associate professor of pathology, Harvard Medical School.

June Machover Reinisch, Ph.D., associate professor of psychology, Rutgers University; Melissa Hines, Ph.D., postdoctoral fellow at UCLA's Brain Research Institute; and John A. McLachlan, developmental toxicologist at the National Institute of Environmental Health Scientists, all took time to assist me, and this project has benefited from their concern.

I would like to give special thanks to Larry McGowan, M.D., director of the Division of Gynecologic Oncology and professor of obstetrics and gynecology at George Washington University Medical Center, Washington, D.C., for helping me obtain scientifically balanced information showing all sides of the DES phenomenon without bias or prejudice. It was truly a relationship of teacher and student, for which I am deeply grateful.

In Great Britain I was assisted by Sir Ralph and Lady Marian Dodds; Peter N. Campbell, director of the Courtauld Institute of Biochemistry, London; Professor Francis Dickens; H. G. Lazell, retired director of the Beecham Group; and others.

My own research needs were ably met by Emily R. Turk, whose great enthusiasm for the project and willingness to constantly find yet another obscure medical publication were of enormous help. I also received research assistance from Jo Ellen Morell and from the wealth of information contained in the doctoral dissertation by Susan Bell. Maura Sughrue, M.D., was kind enough to help me understand the avalanche of material physicians regularly receive. Journalist Eloise Engle, who had begun a DES project of her own, graciously made her files available to me. I would also like to thank John Cary Sims and William B. Schultz of the Public Citizen Litigation Group for their help.

At the Eli Lilly Company, in Indianapolis, I very much appreciated the time spent with me by Raymond Rauch, chief counsel, and Robert H. Furman, the company's current medical director.

From time to time, as I traveled or had a question that needed answering, I was helped by Susan Lebowitz, Peter B. Kovler, Jerold and Helene Sherman, Hilma Lou Ivey, Sandy Danaher, Arnold and Karen York, Arnold Lerman, Anne and Corey Busch, Gunnar and Rosemary Dybwad, Annette Bowling, G. Franklin Rothwell, Daniel Perry, Richard Sughrue, Gary Aldridge, Joe and Lee Cerrell, Michael S. Korney, and Joel Havemann. My parents, Robert T. and Roslyn Meyers, helped me in Los Angeles, and my brother and sister-in-law, Roger and Virginia Meyers, helped me in San Diego.

I wish to acknowledge the friendship and help of several people who helped me complete this manuscript: Ross and Michela Evans generously provided technical assistance that saved me time and anguish. I was also helped by Michael Canyes, Pieter Hartsook, Edward Wolfe, Mary, Diane, and Alice Halsall.

At the beginning of this project Harriet Kramer gave me crucial insights that permitted me to move forward, and Robert Plotkin acted throughout as my unofficial editor, challenging my assumptions, goading me on, and making sensitive and perceptive comments on the manuscript. I cannot thank them enough.

At Seaview/Putnam I benefited from every writer's dream—editors who help a journalist improve his style and concepts. Anne Harrison, Barbara Trainer, and Nancy Perlman worked tirelessly on this book, and the final product is a result of their concern and great talents. My agents, Richard and Arthur Pine, believed in this project from its earliest days, and their help is greatly appreciated.

There were others who helped me on this project, but they did so with the understanding that their names would be withheld. Because of that agreement I cannot thank them publicly now, but their efforts are well remembered.

Alexandria, Virginia
November 4, 1982

For
Karen Marie Sughrue
with love and affection

CONTENTS

1

AN AMERICAN SOCIAL PHENOMENON

DES is a wonder drug that went wrong.

Diethylstilbestrol, the scientific name for DES, is a perfectly legal prescription compound that was widely given by physicians with the best of intentions to millions of American women for more than thirty years in the debatable belief that it would prevent miscarriages.

In the wake of its widespread use in every corner of the country, millions of daughters and sons of the women who took the drug may now find their own hopes of having healthy families compromised and their personal lives changed. Some young women have gotten a rare form of vaginal cancer. Some DES sons, now in their twenties, have gotten testicular cancer. Other women and men may be at a higher risk for other kinds of cancer later in life.

No one knows how many people were exposed to DES from the late 1930s until the early 1970s, but a conservative estimate is six million people, with other estimates going considerably higher. In this country the number of DES-exposed people is at least equal to the entire population of Massachusetts, or Georgia, or Washington state and West Virginia combined. Some experts think the DES population in the country may be as high as ten million.

At least 3 percent of the nation's current population was exposed during pregnancy to a new and apparently miraculous drug that by today's standards hadn't been sufficiently tested. It was continuously marketed for more than three decades in the face of critical animal studies documenting abnormalities in animal offspring, and growing human studies showing it was ineffective in preventing miscarriages. DES came along during the baby boom, an American era of social optimism, when science was king, physicians were often regarded as gods, and drug company salesmen were merchant princes.

The DES phenomenon happened around the world as physicians in other nations, following the American lead, used this wonder drug intended to cure the age-old curse of miscarriages. Other countries have also seen in DES daughters a high incidence of a rare form of vaginal cancer that American scientists have conclusively associated with DES use. But only in America have scientists followed the wide variety of other problems that have since been linked to the use of the drug. Only in America is the DES story an evolving story, as every day seems to bring a new revelation about its chemical impact on the women who took it, the children they bore, and even on their grandchildren. And some children of the drug's users are now finding themselves unsuccessful in their desperate attempts to have children of their own.

The DES story will continue to unfold for the next twenty years at least. It is a story unprecedented in scope, one that affects three generations of Americans.

In 1945 World War II was over, and triumphant soldiers came marching home again, to woo and wed the women of their dreams. Together they would start the world anew. America was changing, on the go; it was witnessing a period of enormous economic growth and social change. Highways swirled out from the cities to the country, transforming farmland into the first suburbs, designed as fine places to raise the kids. In 1947 the first new American car in twenty years, the Kaiser-Frazer, was introduced. From 1945 to 1950 the number of new housing starts went from 326,000 to 1.95 million, a nearly 600 percent increase. In 1945 the Dow Jones Industrial average reached 151, the highest point since the beginning of the war. In 1950 it closed at 235, a 64 percent increase in half a decade.

One primary concern of the returning vets and their sweethearts was the desire to return to the normal business of life. That meant getting married, setting up a household, and having children. As a skinny kid named Frank Sinatra got everybody into a romantic mood, and Burns and Allen kept the chuckles up as the family gathered around the Stromberg-Carlson radio, the marriage rate soared. From about 12 people married per 1,000 during the early 1940s, by 1946 the number skyrocketed to 16.4 per 1,000, as 2.29 million people tied the knot—the highest marriage rate in U.S. history before or since. And with the marriage boom came the baby boom, a phenomenon that would change the way the country lived, worked, and played during the next twenty years of its unprecedented postwar prosperity.

The first wave of the swelling baby tide arrived in 1943, but the birth rate exploded in 1946: 3.4 million children were born, at a rate of 24.1 per 1,000, the highest birth rate since the flapper era prosperity of the 1920s. More than 3.5 million babies were born annually from 1947 to 1953, and more than 4 million were born annually from 1954 to 1964, until the birth rate started to decline in the mid-1960s.

For every four successful pregnancies, however, there has always been one unsuccessful pregnancy—one failure to give birth—which was equally true during a time when having babies was the unofficial national duty, when baby-food makers and diaper services sponsored contests seeking the cutest kiddies, when sometimes it seemed as if every woman in sight was pregnant.

Miscarriages are common, and usually, in the intricate poetry of the human body, logical. Most of them are due to a faulty union between the egg and the sperm, biochemical imbalances, infectious diseases, poor maternal nutrition, abnormal shape and function of the fallopian tubes, uterus, or ovaries, and a host of other factors. A miscarriage, in the simplest sense, is the body's way of stating that a pregnancy "isn't right." Though traumatic and distressing, it often serves a natural and common function in human reproduction.

In this newly modern era of medicine it was realized that many conceptions spontaneously abort before the woman is aware she is pregnant. With that knowledge, the estimated miscarriage rate was raised from 10 percent to 20 percent of all pregnancies. In 1947, for example, there were 3,817,000 live births throughout the country; there were also 954,000 miscarriages. In 1950 there were 3,632,000 live births and an estimated 908,000 miscarriages. Nearly one million miscarriages occurred annually in the era of the baby boom. The need was there for a medicine to prevent this, and the market was there.

Today the use of drugs during pregnancy is in many quarters.taboo. Pregnancy is regarded as too sensitive, too delicate a time to be introducing powerful foreign substances into the body. The women who were pregnant in the postwar American decades and up until the 1960s, however, were among the most medicated women in history. One study conducted between 1958 and 1965 showed that nearly half of them had taken anywhere from two to four pharmaceutical products during their pregnancies. The products ranged from aspirin to tranquilizers to hormones, all of which have since been shown to be potentially harmful to the unborn child. Taking drugs was a part of the national belief system: if America had won two wars overseas, it could win the war on health problems, including miscarriages.

Most women who have a miscarriage will later have a successful pregnancy: in any group of 20 women with miscarriages, perhaps as many as 14 will eventually have children, often with the next attempt. Only a very small number of miscarriages, perhaps 6 out of 20, are due to factors that cannot be corrected with therapy.

It has been that way forever.

But in postwar America, when pregnancy was so avidly sought by so many couples, a miscarriage could be enough to distort a woman's perspective, a family's peace, a couple's dreams. And postwar America turned to science to provide the solution. Medicine had become a new world of miracle drugs, wonder drugs, drugs so new that many of them had not existed a decade or even a year before, drugs so potent they cured—not stopped, but cured—diseases and disabilities once thought unconquerable.

For example, sulfa drugs had been in wide use since 1936. Penicillin had been established as a wonder drug in 1941, killing off bacteria and proving harmless to soldiers in the field. Vitamins, known for years as essential for good health, were widely regarded as another class of miracle drugs, especially after the synthesis in 1947 of vitamin A, and its widespread use as a food additive. Other vitamins—B complex, C, D, E, and K—received widespread attention in the popular press in the 1940s and 1950s as important nutritional aids.

There was no gap between a bustling, optimistic, can-do America and the technical, chemical, and medical aids it used and required in fulfilling its dreams. America was optimistic. At the same time, there was little caution or concern about the use of relatively untested household or medical products either on people or on the world around them—concern that is commonplace today.

Humphrey Bogart giving Ingrid Bergman a world-weary look in the film *Casablanca* had a cigarette dangling from his lips. (An habitual smoker, he died of lung cancer.) Kids stood on goofy-looking X-ray machines when they got fitted for shoes, and years later found out that radiation exposure was potentially harmful. The captains and foot soldiers of industry who owned and worked in America's expanding factories and mills did so without the benefit of antipollution devices.

Postwar America's standards of testing for drugs and other products reflected an era more trusting of people in authority, less concerned about long-term consequences, more sanguine about the close connections between industries and the government that is supposed to regulate them. Today a drug is extensively tested first on animals before it is given to people. Several generations of animals can be tested in the search for long-range effects. Manufacturers must show that not only is a drug safe but also that it is effective. Things were a bit different in the 1940s, however.

There *were* standards, thought to be good at the time but which could hardly pass muster today. The Food and Drug Administration required that any new product must be proven to be safe before it could be marketed. Therefore, drugs were tested—on humans, not animals. When scientists looked for long-range effects, they looked for several months, no more. The objectivity of the tests was considered to be as great as the reputations of those conducting them: the better the reputations, the more reliable the tests. The idea of built-in psychological biases was dismissed as improbable: the concept of controlled, double-blind experiments, today a standard method for eliminating human error, was then controversial. The DES story tragically reflects America's scientific naïveté. The drug was developed with the best of intentions, to answer a serious problem.

One long-established fact is that in the second half of a pregnancy a woman's body needs enormous amounts of progesterone, a natural hormone that the body secretes. During pregnancy, progesterone has a dramatic effect on the cells of the uterus, preparing them to accept and then maintain the growing baby. The baby lives inside the embryonic sac, growing during its nine-month prenatal life from a union of a sperm and an egg to a human organism containing two hundred billion cells. Some miscarriages are due to a lack of progesterone, which causes the endometrium (the inside lining of the womb) to cast out the fertilized ovum.

Before the 1940s the only way to get extra progesterone into the human body was through painful and costly injections. During that decade, however, physicians in the United States began using a new synthetic drug, a miracle drug, in an attempt to prevent miscarriages. The drug, called diethylstilbestrol, produced the same effects as natural estrogens, or female hormones. According to leading scientists, diethylstilbestrol, or DES, could stimulate progesterone. This fact could be measured, they believed, by the appearance of a substance called pregnanediol in the pregnant woman's urine. As will be discussed later in more detail, that would indicate increased levels of progesterone in the bloodstream, so that a normal hormonal environment could be created. If that happened, and many physicians and drug companies claimed that it did, then threatened abortions could be prevented.

There were concerns: all estrogens were known to cause cancer in test animals, and DES, a synthetic laboratory product, was immediately seen to be two or three times more potent than its natural equivalent. Early animal tests with DES showed that it did indeed produce cancerous lesions in some animals. Several articles in technical journals said the offspring of animals treated with DES had structural and anatomic deformities.

But DES was cheap—treatment with it might be as much as three hundred times less expensive than treatment with natural progesterone; it could be taken orally; and, because it was easily manufactured, it could be made widely available. DES was approved by the Food and Drug Administration in 1941 for use in various estrogen-related disorders during and after menopause. Six years later, in 1947, during the height of the baby boom, it was approved for use during pregnancy to prevent miscarriages.

What happened then makes one of the most extraordinary chapters in American medical and social history. DES became the drug of choice in preventing miscarriages despite the doubts about it. It provided doctors with a means to prevent miscarriages rather than having to tell patients there was nothing to be done. It was given to some women who had never been pregnant before; it was given to pregnant women who were experiencing no problems in their pregnancies; it was given to others who had had one or two miscarriages or had had a baby and then a miscarriage. It was given for short periods of time, long periods of time, to women who experienced nausea while taking it, to women who were told they were taking only vitamins.

It was made or distributed by 267 drug companies, which were all able to produce the drug because it was an unpatented generic product. But although its basic chemical formula was always the same, manufacturers added vitamins, other chemicals, or distinctive coatings. One physician in California reportedly made DES pills in his own backroom laboratory. In view of the extreme sensitivity of the fetus to any outside stimulus and the widespread problems that have since been seen in the offspring, it is not known what effects these variations in manufacturing processes might have had.

Millions of American women were given the drug, and they went on to have millions of children. The drug was mainly used in private practice, and the women who took it were mainly white and middle-class.

At the same time that many physicians were dispensing it, other physicians were questioning whether it worked at all. Many of the women to whom DES was given were told to spend most of their pregnancies in bed. A number of researchers began to speculate that these successful deliveries were the result of bed rest and not the drug. By the mid-1950s several impressive studies had been done, showing that DES was a failure: using precise techniques to eliminate their own biases, they marshaled convincing evidence that DES did not prevent miscarriages.

Nevertheless the drug stayed on the market, even after a 1962 change in the law requiring drug manufacturers to show that their products were effective. DES could not pass that test with any certainty, and no one—including the 267 American drug companies that made, marketed, or distributed DES—bothered to try. It even stayed on the market after the thalidomide disaster in the early 1960s. Like DES, thalidomide was given to women during pregnancy, and crossed the placental barrier, once thought to be an almost ironclad defense for the fetus, causing a shocking loss of limbs in offspring.

DES remained a matter of medical dispute until 1971, when several physicians published an article that even in conservative medical terms could be called astounding: DES had been associated by them with a phenomenally rare form of vaginal cancer in young girls born to women who had taken the drug decades earlier during pregnancy. The cancer, called clear-cell adenocarcinoma, had previously been seen only in much older women, usually past the menopause.

The meticulously detailed finding meant that DES had gone from being a miracle drug to the world's first transplacental carcinogen. It crossed the placental barrier and somehow affected the developing cells of the embryo in such a way that vaginal or cervical cancer was discovered ten, twenty, and thirty years later in the daughters of the women who had taken it during pregnancy.

We will never know precisely how many women took DES during pregnancy. In keeping with attitudes regarding the doctor-patient relationship, many women weren't told what they were taking. Others have discovered that the drug wasn't listed on their charts or was listed only as vitamins. Still others have learned that their charts were routinely destroyed, or destroyed in the wake of the DES cancer scare, or that the doctors who treated them have died. And many women have simply forgotten what pills they took decades before. The drug companies may

know, but because of legal considerations they are not revealing their
information; the federal government may know, but if it does, the information has never been compiled anywhere.

The 1971 article linking DES and vaginal cancer set off a great panic
in millions of American mothers and daughters, who feared that a his-
torically unprecedented wave of vaginal cancer was about to strike
young women not yet out of their teens. That type of cancer, if not
caught quickly enough, could kill. Even if caught early, it could require
the surgical removal of the vagina and uterus, eliminating all reproductive capacity, and, with an artificial vagina inserted, reducing sensations
during sexual intercourse. That panic subsided to the level of anxiety as
researchers determined that the rate of vaginal/cervical cancer in DES
daughters is no greater than 1.4 in 1,000, and that the disease has been
diagnosed so far in roughly 400 women.

In the years since the 1971 study, especially in the last years of the
1970s and the first years of the 1980s, new studies on the impact of
DES show that it has caused other enormous disruptions in the bodies
of the children exposed to it *in utero,* when the fetus was no more than
an inch or two long. Although cancer is the most widely known associated effect of DES exposure, it is, in fact, statistically the least significant aspect of it.

Studies show that DES daughters may be at a two to three times
greater risk of having premature babies—in part because of structural
and anatomical differences in their bodies—when compared to women
not exposed to the drug. A premature birth can endanger the baby's
health or even cause its death. DES daughters may face a greater
chance that some of them will never be able to become pregnant, because of changes in their reproductive systems, or may have more difficulty than unexposed women in becoming pregnant. Some studies suggest they may have more menstrual problems and vaginal infections
than unexposed women, although there is some dispute about this in
the field. A number of women interviewed for this book complained
about pain during intercourse, although those findings have not been
seen in the major studies. At least three out of ten—some reports say as
many as nine out of ten—will develop adenosis, a nonmalignant cell
growth in the vagina that apparently goes away with time but that may
be related to vaginal infections and other problems. And there is the
concern that as DES daughters reach menopause they may be at an increased risk for clear-cell adenocarcinoma. A DES daughter, whether
she is a teenager or married woman, must live with that possibility for
the rest of her life.

Some studies suggest that DES sons may be at a greater risk for lowered sperm counts, possibly caused by growths in the testicles which block the flow of sperm. Besides the possibility of impaired fertility, there is also an increased incidence of undescended testicles at birth (which has previously been associated with testicular cancer), as well as cysts inside the sexual organs, and microphallus (small penis).

DES mothers, the women who took the drug, may be at increased risk of breast cancer in a more virulent form and at an earlier age than women who did not take the drug. There is also concern about an increased risk of ovarian cancer and thyroid problems.

For years sex hormones have been known to affect the behavior of laboratory animals. And in this connection, as we shall see later, DES has been shown in several studies to "flavor," or subtly change, the psychological responses of DES children as measured on standard tests, when compared to their own nonexposed siblings.

Even people who never actually took the drug may be at risk for some of its effects, since for decades DES was used across the country as a growth stimulant in cattle, chicken, and sheep. At one point 75 percent of all cattle headed for consumption on the dining tables of America had been raised on DES.

As a result of revelations regarding the drug, a uniquely American recourse has been used by some DES-exposed people: they've gone to court and sued. Lawsuits filed in DES cases in virtually every state in the union seek damages in the billions of dollars and have raised new and important legal questions that could dramatically change the way business is conducted and the law is practiced.

What is a manufacturer's responsibility for a drug's safety? For how long should he be liable? Can damages be collected if a person is hurt by being exposed to a generic (commonly made) product, but can't identify the specific manufacturer? Can an individual collect for the worry he or she endures? Can damages be collected decades after the exposure?

In response to some of the verdicts that went against them, manufacturers are asking their state and federal legislators to pass laws overriding court decisions. The insurance industry is heavily involved. Like the impact of the drug itself, the results of all this legal and legislative activity will not be known for years.

The scope of the DES nightmare is only beginning to be understood. By virtue of its medical impact on so many people in so many ways, and its social impact on the medical, legal, and governmental professions, it has become one of the most influential and destructive health products in the twentieth century. By comparison:

- The drug thalidomide is widely known to have caused deformities in children whose pregnant mothers took it as a tranquilizer: babies were born with flippers instead of arms and legs. Thalidomide was most widely used in Europe; rarely used in the United States, and an estimated 8,000 children, most of whom were born outside the United States, were affected.
- Toxic Shock Syndrome, associated with tampon use, has harmed at least 2,000 women, of whom more than 130 have died, with an estimated 50 new cases reported each month.
- Since 1970 more than 1.1 million women have suffered from acute pelvic infections as a result of using intrauterine devices (IUDs). As many as one in four is or will be sterile because of such use.

But the millions of women and men who are DES-exposed are still coming of age, and many of them, like others in the country, have put off for social reasons trying to have a child now. They may not know for years how their fertility has been affected. Any changes in the body that occur over time—such as vaginal cancer after menopause—may not become evident for years. It is an unparalleled situation.

There is no such thing as a safe drug. We know that today, in a less optimistic, more critical time than the one that came in with the Levittowns and Uncle Miltie and the June Taylor Dancers. DES, a legal and tested drug yesterday, has turned dreams into nightmares today. There were early reports of its toxicity, concerns in the medical profession about its misuse, studies showing it did not work. Yet it was marketed and sold and used for more than thirty years in this country—a bitter pill swallowed by women who wanted only babies, who wanted only the best that life in America had to offer.

2
THREE FAMILIES

Eva Schwartz, Virginia Childs, and Mary Brown have never met one another, but they are linked by a bond almost as strong as the mother-hood they have in common. Each woman wanted a baby more than twenty-five years ago, each had the common experience of a previous miscarriage, each consulted her doctor, each took dozens of a tiny white pill, and each gave birth to a loved and wanted child.

The pill was DES, and the impact on the lives of their children, their families, and on them is still being felt, years after the event itself.

The DES story has many aspects, but it is preeminently a story of people—the women who took it, the children born to them, the hus-bands and wives and mothers and fathers who live with the knowledge of problems today and potential problems tomorrow. All the other as-pects—the laboratory calculations, the clinical testing, the economic marketing, the government regulation—are really elements that enter the funnel of American health care and come out on the doorsteps of American consumers.

The three families in this chapter represent a broad spectrum of DES-exposed people. Their experiences show, as no cold statistic can, the evolving knowledge about DES exposure, and how that knowledge, aside from any medical complications, can alter and change lives.

Boston native Eva Schwartz, for example, read in 1971 about the startling association between DES and clear-cell adenocarcinoma in daughters exposed during pregnancy. Her daughter Andrea was imme-diately examined, and no cancer was found. In 1976 and 1980, how-ever, Andrea had ectopic pregnancies, pregnancies lodged in the fallopian tubes instead of in the uterus. Both fallopian tubes were removed. At that time no statistical association had been made in any study of DES daughters showing that they were at a higher risk for ectopic pregnancies than anyone else. In 1981 the association was made known publicly.

Virginia Childs took DES in Philadelphia. Her daughter Carla has had two healthy children. But she had them sooner than she and her husband thought they would have to. They decided to start their family because they didn't know what the future would bring—specifically, whether it would bring vaginal cancer and the possible surgical removal of her vagina or cervix. In 1975 Carla knew she had unusual ridges on her cervix but had no way of knowing what that meant. In 1981 a medical paper for the first time associated the presence of those cervical ridges with adverse pregnancy outcomes such as premature births and miscarriages.

In Oakland, California, Mary Brown took pills to prevent a miscarriage, and spent an adult lifetime worrying about her son Gary's physical development and reproductive capacity. Like many other DES mothers, she has been unable to get her own medical records. Many of the problems Gary has developed are precisely those experienced by other men with confirmed DES exposure, and they are problems not associated with any other pregnancy medications except DES. The initial information on DES-exposed children dealt only with daughters and vaginal cancer—trying enough for women whose daughters had problems that were not cancer-related. But Mary's child was a boy, and no one talked at all about DES sons until the late 1970s. The federal government's first report on DES sons is scheduled for late 1983, twelve years after DES first came to public attention. Because of federal funding cutbacks, it may well be the last government report on sons.

The DES-exposed people in this country, millions of them, lived with fears for the future based on their own anecdotal knowledge of the subject. Attempts to learn more were frustrated by a lack of precise information and reluctance on the part of some physicians to give them what information was available.

Information seesaws back and forth across one great fulcrum—knowledge. If a woman does not know she is DES-exposed, she cannot seek special medical treatment. If she knows she is DES-exposed, and a physician denies she is at any great risk, she may be unprepared. Even if she knows she is exposed and takes precautions, it is possible that as-yet unstudied aspects of DES exposure may interfere with her life or with the child-bearing process. DES was a drug that had outraced the ability of science to keep it in check; the DES-exposed population outraced the scientific community in knowledge of its problems. Scientific knowledge is based on precise information; personal knowledge is based on monthly menstrual cycles and daily showers; the gap can be filled with fear.

The members of the three families in this chapter started out with raw personal knowledge, and they have since modified it as the scientific information has been revealed. The wait, for some of them, was a long time coming. Their stories, told in the context of their families, with kids gathered around, toys on the carpet, or family photos on the table, is a good introduction to this remarkable American social phenomenon.

During the Second World War, before her marriage, Eva Schwartz worked in a defense plant where aircraft parts were made. After her June 19, 1945, marriage she stopped work to stay at home, keep house, and shortly afterward, care for her first child—a son, Michael, born at the start of the boom, on April 26, 1946. Her husband, a photographer of children, supported the family.

In 1953, when she was pregnant with her daughter Andrea, she converted the dining room of her three-decker suburban Boston apartment into a bedroom for the coming baby. One bedroom was already occupied by her seven-year-old son, and Mrs. Schwartz and her husband had the other bedroom. The growing family needed more room, and the dining room conversion was the only choice.

To keep warm in the freezing Boston winters, she said, "I got up at five A.M. every morning to shovel coal—that's what you had to do in those days. The coal furnace was in the cellar. Later it was converted to oil. In the kitchen we cooked on a stove with a five-gallon oil tank attached. It seems crazy now, shoveling coal like that, but when you're young, it's fun."

Between the birth of her son and the pregnancy with her daughter Mrs. Schwartz became pregnant twice, but each pregnancy ended in a miscarriage. When she got pregnant again, in early 1953, she felt this would be the last time. "I was in my mid thirties, and I felt this was it. I decided to have a child no matter what." When she experienced some spotting early in pregnancy, her doctor gave her a drug to take to prevent a miscarriage. She took it, under doctor's orders, every day for nearly seven months.

The drug was diethylstilbestrol, or DES. And every day she took it she felt nauseated.

"I was sick every day. As soon as I'd eat, I'd heave again. I spent much of the time in bed. I wanted to die. During my first pregnancy, with Michael, there had been no problems at all. I was healthy as a horse. And when I stopped taking the drug, at the end of the seventh month, with Andrea, I felt reborn."

Nausea and vomiting experienced by women who took DES were common side effects seen by drug company researchers and practicing physicians during the 1940s, when DES was being tested. No one knew exactly why some women had these reactions and others didn't, although it was evident that the larger the dosage, the more violent the reaction. The reactions, however, were not regarded as clinically significant and were discounted by drug company scientists, doctors, and federal regulatory officials, who were more impressed by its apparent ability to prevent miscarriages.

Eva Schwartz's daughter Andrea was born on September 27, 1953. "When she was a little girl she was very chubby. I read an article in the paper about DES, that it was being used in poultry to fatten them up. I said to my husband, 'Maybe that's why she's so chubby.' " She sighs. "On top of making me sick, look what it did to my daughter."

Andrea Schwartz Goldstein is now 29 years old. As was mentioned earlier, she has lost both fallopian tubes following two ectopic pregnancies. Her uterus is severely misshapen, the apparent cause of a third failed pregnancy, this one an intrauterine pregnancy (occurring inside the uterine cavity). The precise causes are unknown. What *is* known about Andrea Goldstein, her parents, her husband, and their adopted son, Jarrod, is the constant pain and emotional anguish she has suffered.

"My mother told me I was exposed when the first reports came out in 1971," she said. "The first gynecologist I went to, in 1971, just told me to get a Pap smear every six months [a standard method for determining the health of the cervix and vagina]. The second one, in 1973, told me the same thing. The third one, in 1975, said, 'Do you realize you have a pinhole opening in your cervix?' I said, 'No.' "

She is amazed. "What happened to the first two doctors? Why did they miss that?" She pauses, adjusting some of the papers in front of her, the road maps to her problems. "I got married in 1975 and pregnant in 1976, and on Veterans Day I woke up in considerable pain, with heavy bleeding. It turned out to be my first ectopic pregnancy, on my left fallopian tube, which was then removed."

After two years' effort, she became pregnant again. "It didn't feel like a good pregnancy. You know that expression 'A woman knows'? I knew. I feared it was another ectopic, but it was in the uterus, and of course it didn't last. That pregnancy would have been twins. In 1980, after two years of trying, I got pregnant for the third time, and when I went into the hospital because of the pain, I knew I risked losing my remaining tube. In surgery, because of the hemorrhaging, it was either the tube or me. All of this has given me a mid-life crisis in my twenties."

Before her third surgery—during which her remaining fallopian tube was removed, thus eliminating all possibility of pregnancy—Andrea and Paul Goldstein tried mightily to have a child.

"When a couple is trying to get pregnant," Andrea said, "one of the things you do is have intercourse whether you want to or not. You're not thinking of sensual relations at all. You're blinded. Now we look back and see what a perverse situation it was."

Paul agreed. "At times it made quite a difference. My wife would get quite uptight, depressed, and bummed out by the fact she couldn't get pregnant. But it also reaches the point of no return. I love my wife, I feel for my wife, but if that's the way it is, you make the best of what you have."

During the four years of her life when she was trying to have a baby, Andrea found herself increasingly isolated from other women her age who had children. "I lost my friends. They had babies—I couldn't hack it. I went to see a psychiatrist. That helped somewhat. But it's hard to be with people who have children when you can't. I started to remember things from my childhood. When I was about five I remember holding my cousin and saying, 'When I grow up I want to have a baby.' But suddenly I was losing control of my dreams. We bought a house in 1976, thinking we'd have a baby there, but ten weeks later I had my first operation. I'd go to shopping malls and be okay until I'd see women with babies. I became struck by the fact that I'd never be a grandmother. I didn't want a gold medal in the Olympics, I wanted a baby. Some flowers can reproduce asexually. I can't reproduce at all."

Andrea and Paul decided to adopt a baby and fulfill their dreams of parenthood that way.

"We found Jarrod, but even that was a problem. It seemed so unfair that because my body wasn't working right we had to be scrutinized by a social worker. But I can't get over not having had the nine-month pregnancy experience. I don't blame my mother at all. I blame the doctors—and the drug companies for making and selling something without enough testing which at the very least was known to be carcinogenic [in animals]."

She has translated her anger into legal action and is involved in a lawsuit in Massachusetts against the companies she claims acted improperly. She is also head of her state chapter of DES Action, a consumer group.

The fertility problems that plagued Andrea Goldstein's waking moments also torment her when she is asleep. In a letter to me after our face-to-face meeting she wrote: "Another disturbing result of my infertility are my frequent (though at this point less frequent) recurrent dreams in which I appear pregnant to everyone but know that I am not. It was some time since one of these occurred, but one did the night after I spoke with you."

Andrea Goldstein's eyes glisten with a rare kind of fury. At the end of our meeting, on a chilly gray October afternoon, she walked me to the door of her office, located not far from the hospitals in Boston where DES had been tested on people and found to be safe and effective for use during pregnancy. Two gold medals dangled around her neck: one was engraved "12-9-79," the date of her son's birth, and the other "1-28-80," the day she and Paul took their son home.

She said to me, "I know that the last thought I have before I die will be that I never had the experience of giving birth."

Virginia Childs was a young bride in the mid-1940s when she and her husband moved to Philadelphia. Jack had just gotten out of the Navy, and, like the rest of America, the Childses were intent on putting the war behind them and starting an independent life. Married in 1944, Mrs. Childs had had a miscarriage, then a son, Norris, and then a second miscarriage before becoming pregnant with her second child. A daughter named Carla was born in 1948.

Those were heady times for young Americans. Television was such a new phenomenon that *Life* magazine ran a map showing the states that had stations, and by 1949, one hundred thousand TV sets were being sold each week. Viewers and readers were urged to figure out "Which Twin Has the Toni?" Walter Winchell tapped out his gossip and news to Mr. and Mrs. America and all the ships at sea, and if you really wanted a terrific smile, you'd pick up some Ipana toothpaste from the corner druggist.

"It was a different era," recalled John N. (Jack) Childs, Jr., Virginia's husband and Carla's father. "We were a conquering nation home from 'war. A lot of mistakes could be made, but they were not fatal ones. People today look at the world differently, more cautiously."

Unlike in her earlier miscarriage, Mrs. Childs experienced no pregnancy problems with Carla, who was born on September 16, 1948.

"There was no staining and no spotting with her. But I had had an ovarian cyst removed in 1945, and I had endometriosis [abnormal glands and supportive tissue which have moved from their normal place in the lining of the womb, a not unusual development in some women]. I was given the pills to help me keep the baby."

Although Mrs. Childs had experienced two miscarriages before she became pregnant with Carla, there were no medical indications in that pregnancy for DES to be used. There was nothing to indicate that the pregnancy was not a healthy one. As we will see in later chapters, the language of various medical papers advocating DES use sometimes gets fuzzy: DES was recommended in cases of actual threatened abortion (the older term for what today are called miscarriages) or to prevent threatened abortion. This confusion of language was implicitly encouraged by various drug companies, which were out to sell a product. One east coast company, the Grant Chemical Company of Brooklyn, even recommended in one ad that DES be used as a preventive measure in *all* pregnancies.

It was being used by Mrs. Childs's doctor as a precaution.

DES was completely forgotten by Virginia Childs for twenty-seven years, until Carla, then a Radcliffe College graduate and Peace Corps veteran of Nukualofa, Tonga, in the South Pacific, was undergoing a routine gynecological examination in Philadelphia.

"I was on the [examining] table, and the doctor said, 'Hmmm, did your mother take any drugs when she was pregnant with you?' My first thought was cancer!" Carla Childs remembers.

Virginia Childs didn't know, and she had no records of her own to consult. When she called her gynecologist, the nurse assured her that she had not taken DES during her pregnancy. But Carla was exhibiting adenosis, unusual tissue in the vagina and cervix, which was then commonly interpreted as evidence that cancer was on the way.

"Carla *needed* those records, and when I called the nurse, she said they had been sent to her doctor. But they never arrived. Finally I went to my physician's office, and the nurse went over the records again, and in fact they *did* show that I had taken DES with her. The nurse made all these excuses—'Oh, the doctor's handwriting's so hard to read,' she said. When I talked to the doctor about it, he shrugged it off. 'Millions of pregnant women were given the drug. Only a few girls get cancer,' he said casually. Although I'd gone to him since 1946, I immediately switched doctors," Virginia Childs said with conviction.

"The drug appeared to be the best medical practice at the time," Jack Childs said in his gravelly, businessman's voice. "I don't have strong feelings one way or the other about the fact that she took it. But I was disturbed at the doctor's brushing her off. That was inexcusable."

Virginia Childs added: "I don't feel guilty. I wanted the baby. Maybe I'm wrong in not feeling guilty, but I wanted another child."

Carla's examining physician had also seen some cervical ridges, another common development in DES daughters, and recommended that Carla go to a DES center at the hospital of the University of Pennsylvania, in Philadelphia, where she was studying for a master's degree.

"In the space of one year I had twelve gynecological exams. There were a lot of biopsies [the removal of tissue for microscopic examination]. The biopsies were done without anesthesia, and they hurt. They pinched. When I got an abnormal Pap smear, I was told to come in the following week, because there was a threat of cancer, and that weekend I invited all my friends to come over for a party. I was glad when no one came. I was in tears the whole weekend."

The Pap smear indicated that more examination was required, although it did not specifically suggest cancer. But Carla remembers this: "When I got the bad Pap smear I said, 'Take it out! take it out! There's this terrible thing in me! When in doubt, take it out!' But the doctors said no."

She was lucky they did, because other women in the same circumstances have undergone partial vaginectomies (removal of part or all of the vagina) from activist physicians practicing what was then regarded by some as proper medical response to the perceived cancer threat indicated by adenosis. A woman's ability to have children can be altered or eliminated by such a procedure, depending upon how much of the vagina is removed. Today the practice of partial vaginectomies in those circumstances is widely regarded as an overreaction to a medical condition that usually goes away with time, and is viewed by many feminists as an example of how male physicians freely operate on female patients.

. Carla had another macabre experience when she sought mental health counseling for her cancer fears at the student health center. She asked for an immediate appointment to "talk out" her problems and was told that she could have an immediate appointment only if she was suicidal.

"I told them I didn't want to *die,* I wanted to *live.*" She didn't get the appointment.

Carla had just begun a relationship with a young urban planner named Bill Cozzens, whom she later married. The agony of the DES exposure brought them closer together. "Bill was the shoulder for me," she said. "I felt it was totally unfair, that it shouldn't have to happen to me. The prospect of losing my uterus was a wipeout. I couldn't tell anyone about it except my parents and Bill, and they were supportive."

Bill's experience was not without pain, however. He recalled: "At the time we were just beginning our relationship, and we were at that stage where you're still evaluating whether you want to stay with someone or not. I recall thinking that Carla really didn't have cancer, but then I hadn't read much about it. There was some distancing going on, some reassessing. I wasn't saying, 'Don't burden me,' but also in some corner of my mind I was reassessing the relationship."

Their experience is typical of those first young couples trying to deal with DES exposure, especially its all-too-many unknown aspects. Now in various parts of the country there are counseling groups, support sessions, hot lines, and informative pamphlets. But none of these existed back in the dark ages of the 1970s. In fact, one of the earliest papers advising physicians on how to deal with DES-exposed people was published only in 1977.

Carla did not develop cancer, but after their marriage in 1977 she and Bill began thinking about children, before they had ever thought they would have to—another indication of the way that DES has shaped untold numbers of American lives.

"Use it before you lose it," Carla said she had thought philosophically.

"I don't think we would have tried to actively get pregnant if it hadn't been for that bad Pap smear," Bill said recently. As we talked in their Maryland home, Carla nursed their three-month-old son Daniel as three-year-old Jean played in the background.

"Getting pregnant was no problem, but during my second month with Jean there was bleeding, and my only feelings were panic, panic, panic. Daniel was also planned, and there was bleeding in the second month with him too. I stayed in bed for the last three weeks, fearing a premature delivery"—a common experience of DES daughters, as other women will relate in this book. Ironically enough, had Carla been born twenty years earlier, a well-meaning doctor might have given her DES for the bleeding during her pregnancies.

While she was at the University of Pennsylvania, Carla's worries about her own DES exposure prompted her to organize a consumer group, which later became part of the national consumer group, DES Action. She posted hand-lettered signs on trees and bulletin boards. At the first meeting eighteen DES daughters showed up.

Consumers' groups have flourished in many fields when individuals have been unable to get information, sympathy, support, and friendship from professionals. In the absence of facts, the groups often serve the purpose of helping people keep their wits about them as they search for answers, and reinforce the idea that they are not alone.

"It was great. Many of us had had the same thoughts: Oh, I'm going crazy, I can't handle it, I ought to get pregnant even without a husband. The *fears* of someone who doesn't have cancer can be worse than cancer, because no one will give you information. In the first throes of knowing you were exposed, it's hard to think you will ever get beyond it, but you do. There's always the concern now whether I'll be more cancer-prone. There's a history of cancer in our family, so I expect cancer to be a factor in my life, regardless of DES. But I don't ever want to forget the fear and trauma I went through, even though I am now beyond it," she said.

The same optimism and excitement about life that the Schwartz and Childs families felt on the east coast was also felt in the West.

"Oakland was a really nice place to grow up and live in," recalled Mary Rossi Brown, sitting in her comfortable living room with her husband, Lloyd, a dentist, and their second son, Gary, the sales manager for a regional forklift company. "Most of the people who had grown up here still lived here. Everyone knew everyone else. When we wanted an 'occasion' we went into San Francisco, across the Bay. We always wore hats and gloves, because it was something special."

In 1944 Lloyd and Mary Brown had their first child, and then Mrs. Brown had a miscarriage several years after that. In early 1948 Mary became pregnant with Gary, and during a routine examination at her doctor's office "he gave me some pills. I always wondered why. I didn't want the doctor to give me pills, and later when I asked him, after we knew so much, he said he had given them to me to prevent a miscarriage. I trusted him," she said.

Unlike Mrs. Schwartz and Mrs. Childs, Mary Brown has not been able to find medical records showing that in fact she took DES during her pregnancy. But years later, shortly before he died, the physician acknowledged to her that he had given her pills to prevent a miscarriage. However, when she first became concerned about her son's health, she had difficulty finding a doctor who would pay serious attention to her.

In her desperate search to get answers, in her refusal to accept the bland assurances of the medical establishment, and her endless fear and concern for her child, even after he had entered adulthood and had his own children, Mary Brown is as typical as any other DES-exposed mother. The courage and decency her son and daughter-in-law have shown are also typical of people involved with the DES phenomenon.

"Shortly after he was born I noticed that his penis appeared to be small, and so did one testicle. I thought it was undescended. I took him to a pediatrician, who told me I was wrong, that everything was okay, although to me there still seemed to be something different."

She paused for breath as we sat in her living room, looking to her son and husband for support. Like the other mothers and their children, the flow of words can sometimes get painfully clogged.

"Gary was thin and wiry as a boy, when all of a sudden at age nine he gained weight, a lot of weight. He became very heavy through the hips and neck, and very sluggish and very slow-moving and thinking. I changed doctors, from the pediatrician back to the family doctor. He took one look at him and said his testicle was undescended, that his hormones were out of balance. He made this evaluation on a visual examination in his office. Every time I see pictures of Gary from that time, when he was heavy, I could kill that doctor. Not the one who gave the DES, but the one who said there was nothing wrong."

DES is a synthetic female estrogen, a female sex hormone, and there is some speculation in the medical community that it causes an imbalance in the developing baby's body chemistry. Estrogens in general are known to do this. Exactly why it happens with some young men and not with others is unclear; it may have to do with the precise moment it is given. Today the medical community uses the term "target organ" to specify which organ a drug will affect. It is now know that DES affects the sexual and reproductive tracts.

To correct the perceived imbalance the family doctor prescribed androgen (male hormone) shots, as well as thyroid shots and thyroxine pills. "He said if we had waited a few more years it would have been too late. Now it could be corrected in a matter of weeks," Mary Brown recalled. Gary's father administered the shots at home to the boy, who sometimes cringed in pain.

"I knew the shots were for his benefit," Lloyd Brown said. "But when it's your own kid you hate to hurt him."

"Almost overnight," Gary's mother recalled, "within a few months, the weight problem disappeared, the testicle descended, and his grades went up. We thought, we hoped, the problem was over, but I always wondered, Why did this happen? Was it genetic, the medicine, or what? But that wasn't all, because the doctor who prescribed the shots said if his testicle hadn't descended, he wouldn't have had male tendencies. I was so relieved when he had a girlfriend."

Years later Mrs. Brown took Gary to a university endocrinologist for further tests, to make sure there were no other problems. "He said Gary would be normal but he would never be any taller, that if it hadn't been for this, he would have been six feet tall or more." Gary Brown is five feet nine inches tall. "And that irritated me, the manipulation of my life. They had no right," he said.

In between the early medical exams and the point of maturity at which he fell in love, married, and began raising his own family, the Brown family went through "the living hell" (his mother's phrase) of seeking answers and getting blank stares, of asking questions and getting shrugs.

"The doctors were making my mother think she was crazy. She was dragging me everywhere, I didn't know what was going on. In one doctor's office there were these engineering-style drawings of my testicles, with measurements. As a kid I was always being poked at, having to pull my pants down. It was humiliating."

Once Mary Brown called a radio talk show host, seeking answers. She got no more from the dulcet-toned announcer than she got from most medical authorities. "What about men? Will he be sterile? What about cancer? What about the future? The only answers I got were, 'I don't know, we don't know.' "

In the early 1970s she read an article in one of the women's magazines describing the association between DES use in pregnancy and a rare form of vaginal cancer occurring years later in daughters. "I thought, I bet that's what caused Gary's problem. If it did something to girls, maybe it did something to boys. But I couldn't get any answers. It was my private hell. The whole time I'd wake up in the middle of the night, wondering. I just kept praying a lot."

There were arguments at home between Lloyd (a medical professional himself) and his wife over medical advice given by professional friends of his whose judgment he respected. "When the first doctor said there was nothing wrong, I argued with Lloyd about whether that doctor was right. After all, he was a personal friend of the family."

"In the beginning I was on the spot," Lloyd said. "The doctor was on the same floor as I was. I took his word for it, though I felt there was something radically wrong. I worried, but she worried more. After the second doctor said there was a problem, whenever she took him to someone, she'd come home and we'd discuss it. I'd bring home medical journals from the office, the ones that started to have articles about DES in them. There should have been some real facts available, but there weren't."

Through school Gary kept his fears to himself, worked on his grades, avoided sports because of the body weight he couldn't lose even through relentless dieting, and became more of a recluse than he wanted to be.

"I didn't hang out at Seventh and Wood and pick up tomatoes with the other guys, because I was afraid I was different. That led me into other things. We lived up in the hills, up by ourselves, and I worked with my hands, worked on electricity and plumbing, worked on cars. Now there's *nothing* I can't do," he said with fierce pride.

"When I was younger, living at home, I acted like I didn't care, but deep down I did. When Mom gave me things to read, I pretended to ignore them, but then I went off and read them. At first there was this idea that there was something different about me. Then I realized it wasn't me, that it had been the medicine. When I first gained all that weight, at age nine, I was very conscious of it. You don't like being called Fatso. As a maturing man you're always aware of your body and the fear that somehow I was different. It affects your personality," he said.

"I felt bad that Mom was doing all this for me. I could see by her concern that something was wrong, although I know now she wasn't telling me everything. When I was on the hormone shots I was very nervous, and that was supposed to correct the heaviness! I always tried to avoid the subject. I know she was concerned, she wanted answers, never stopped asking questions, and she was frustrated because she wasn't getting any."

After his marriage Mary Brown wondered about her son's fertility. There had still been no direct conversation between them about possible fertility risks, since most of the information she had gathered concerned cancer in women. But two years after the wedding, with no difficulty at all, his wife Margaret became pregnant with the first of their children.

"During the pregnancy I kept feeling, I hope the child's normal.

Who knew about what would happen? The baby was born, and I secretly went over to check him out. I was delighted, everything was fine," Grandma Brown said.

Gary grinned. "I knew I didn't have to worry about finding out, because she would first."

Margaret added: "If we had had a fertility problem I would have been upset. I really wanted children. We probably would have adopted. Now we're concerned about Gary's health, that he go in for checkups. I do some reading on the subject, mainly from the magazines, but I know it's deeply concerning to him. He must worry about it all the time, although he doesn't say anything. I really didn't know anything about DES until his mother told me that she had been worried all through our pregnancy. Gary is a wonderful husband and father."

After the birth of her grandchild, Mary Brown told her son for the first time all of the information she had accumulated. "I told him to always be checked. He thought it was silly."

That was Gary's public face. This is the private one: "I think I avoid medical checkups because I'm afraid of cancer. No, it's deeper than that: I'm afraid of death, I've always been afraid of death, and I think it comes from all those trips to the doctors when I was a boy. I try to organize my paper work, try to keep everything in order. Deep down I'd like another child, I really love them. Usually you say, 'Well, I can have one in another year,' but what if there are problems with me, what if I can't then, what if I'm dead? Believe me, this kind of thing affects every aspect of your life, your life-style, and your personality."

Three different families—the Schwartzes, the Childses, the Browns. Three different stories, but really only the tip of the iceberg.

3

SIR EDWARD CHARLES DODDS
AND THE SYNTHESIS OF DES

The red doubledecker London buses are a blur a few blocks away on Oxford Street. One block over, the King and Queen pub sells pints of bitter to the medical students and researchers who stop in after rounds at Middlesex Hospital, located at the oddly cramped corner of Riding House and Cleveland streets. Attached to the hospital by a symbolic bridge is the Courtauld Institute of Biochemistry, whose founding director was the man who synthesized DES in 1938, Sir Edward Charles Dodds.

Two American medical scholars and physicians, Kenneth L. Noller and Charles R. Fish, pointed out in a study of DES called "Diethylstilbestrol Usage: Its Interesting Past, Important Present, and Questionable Future," that "A history of the most significant sex hormone research . . . (beginning in the mid-1930's), is a history of one man, E. C. Dodds."

Dodds was a remarkable twentieth-century man, a retail shoe salesman's son who earned both an M.D. degree and a Ph.D. in biochemistry in the same year, 1925. A lover of wines, who quoted Horace's *Odes* learned during his schoolboy years at Harrow, he shocked the uppercrust world of British science by doing consulting work with large drug companies. Behind his back he was called "E. Commercial Dodds" for his efforts and the money he received.

Sir Charles, who insisted that his friends call him Charlie, was about five foot seven, stocky in build, wore tortoiseshell glasses, and in later life was distinguished by a large bald dome and slick black hair at the sides. He loved to race around London in a Rolls-Royce to one of the three or four private clubs in which he held memberships. If he wasn't expounding on chemical structures and new pharmaceutical derivatives, he might be talking about the acid level of wines.

"When he got an idea, he would suddenly start drawing benzene rings on the napkins in restaurants," his son, Sir Ralph Dodds, recalled. Esme Barron, his longtime secretary, who kept his books and handled his globe-trotting travel schedule, remembers him as "a good all-rounder."

Born just before the turn of the century, on October 13, 1899, he had a lively mind that leaped from subject to subject. Although eloquent in his writing and in conversation with friends, he was painfully shy in the laboratories of the Institute, jingling the coins in his pocket until one of his awed students or a professor broke the ice. In the course of his long career, which ended only with his death in 1973, he worked in such fields as endocrinology, penicillin research, and vitamin supplements for food. He published 281 articles in forty-eight years.

Sir Charles's great work was in endocrinology, the study of how and why the body secretes certain chemicals, a field that really began only one or two scientific generations before his birth. Dodds and endocrinology became famous and important together, and the development of DES sprang directly from the man and his field.

A brief history of endocrinology before Dodds can be gleaned from the Noller and Fish article published in the July 1974 issue of *Medical Clinics of North America.* The field started formally in 1874, when a British researcher, Sir William Gull, demonstrated the framework of internal secretions. This preliminary work was concerned with thyroid-gland extracts, but interest in the field quickly shifted to gonadal, or sex, hormones, following long-standing interest in the way the reproductive capacity of the human species works.

During the early part of the twentieth century researchers refined their knowledge as they zeroed in on the delicate chemicals in the body. In 1912 a German researcher, L. Adler, published a paper on the physiology and pathology of ovarian function. A decade later American researcher R. T. Frank began writing papers on the relationship between endocrinology and gynecological functions, specifically showing that the biologically active substance Adler had been talking about was actually a component of a complex fluid inside the ovary rather than the entire ovary itself.

In 1923, American scientists Edgar Allen and Edward A. Doisy, having experimented with test animals, published a paper in the *Journal of the American Medical Association* reporting on the exact location of ovarian hormones, their extraction, and their purification.

Four years later the race for knowledge of female sex hormones speeded up again when German scientists Aschheim and Zondek published their significant finding that pregnant women (not test animals) excrete what is called an estrus-exciting hormone in their urine. That brought science closer to the secrets of what happens (or doesn't happen) during pregnancy and enabled others to work out a test to predict when a woman had gotten pregnant. As the decade of the 1920s was ending, Edward Charles Dodds was lecturing, teaching, and researching at Middlesex Hospital, while the Americans Allen and Doisy were preparing a nearly pure estrogen compound.

About the same time, Dodds's colleague and biographer, Francis Dickens, recalled, "Dodds had the idea that you ought to be able to make artificial substances in the laboratory, free from impurities, to produce the full effects of the natural hormones."

"Dodds was bright, he got the idea that one should apply chemistry to medical diagnosis," said Peter N. Campbell, the current director of the Courtauld Institute of Biochemistry. "He was quite unlike any American figure at the time. To the medical man he was a biochemist; to the biochemist he was a medical man."

In 1928 Charles Dodds was appointed to head up the new Courtauld Institute of Biochemistry, a part of Middlesex Hospital, where he had been the youngest professor ever appointed and the school from which he had received both his advanced degrees. His son, Sir Ralph Dodds, recalls that the Institute had really been set up so that his father could continue his experimental work. He had his office on the fourth floor, his laboratories on the fifth and sixth floors. With his dual specialties in both biochemistry and medicine, he was one of the best qualified people in the world to work on the complex subject of endocrinology.

His reputation for accurate speculative concepts was growing. Several years after Canadian researchers Banting and Best had developed insulin for use in diabetes, Dodds and Francis Dickens developed a new procedure for preparing insulin from the pancreas of oxen, which they personally collected from London slaughterhouses. That marked the first extraction of insulin in Great Britain, Peter Campbell said.

When he was twenty-eight years old, in 1928, Dodds's growing reputation in the field of clinical biochemistry was such that he was called in as a consultant to the ailing King George V. Shortly afterward he was made a Member of the Victorian Order, a signal honor whose initials, M.V.O., he often signed after his name.

According to the article by Noller and Fish, Dodds and his staff produced the world's first artificial estrogen in 1934 and continued to work on its modification for several years. Their products were technically interesting but not very strong, and could be used only through injection. Additionally, it was clear that for commercial application the cost would be prohibitive.

There is no secret as to why the field of endocrinology was attracting the interest of leading scientists around the world. The ability to "get inside" the chemical system of a functioning body, whether a woman's body or an animal's, might have important applications for growth and reproduction. If there were other "female" troubles caused by a lack of a naturally produced sex hormone, then replacing it might help. Female breast cancer and prostate cancer in men were then believed to have a relationship with the body's natural supply of female estrogen or the lack of it. The development of a replacement might help. There might also be other uses for a cheap, active synthetic hormone.

Science has always proceeded in two directions. Scientific medicine refines substances and sketches theories; clinical medicine applies those theories to human life. The intent is always to improve life; the application is determined only after comparing the potential benefit with the potential risk.

Animal work was already showing what some of these products could do: female rats that had had their ovaries removed showed full estrus, or sexual receptivity, after injection with the artificial hormones; and capons, or castrated male chickens, showed female plumage and coloration after similar injections.

"Dodds was always obsessed with finding another key for the lock, the lock being the estrus cycle in animals and sexual development in people," recalled eighty-two-year-old Francis Dickens, who now lives in his retirement cottage in Ferring, ninety minutes from London, where the scent of roses mixes with the breeze from the sea. "He had two phrases he used repeatedly: 'Find the key to the lock,' and 'Simplify, simplify.' "

Dodds wanted to see if the chemical reactions of estrogens could be obtained with a substance that had a chemical base different from the natural substances. This is what he meant by "Simplify, simplify." Scientifically it is a daring and novel approach, one that was being attempted without success elsewhere around the world.

Dodds collaborated with Sir Robert Robinson, who headed Oxford University's Dyson Perrins Laboratory, in an attempt to make the simple compound. The Oxford group had also been working in this field and was well aware that other groups, especially German clinicians, were striving to conquer the field of sex hormones.

The Dodds and Robinson groups formally joined forces in 1938. After a chemist from the Dodds group, Wilfred Lawson, scribbled a new formulation on the back of an envelope, a young student at Oxford, Leon Golberg, performed the actual synthesis of diethlystilbestrol by heating one gram of a similar substance to 205 degrees centigrade. For years the original specimen of DES, now officially a member of the alkyl-substituted dihydroxystilbene family, rested in Lawson's possession.

The substance, always called stilbestrol in England, was quickly perceived to be three times more powerful than naturally occurring estrogen. In addition, it was shown to be orally effective: it could either be taken in a liquid form, diluted in water, or as a pill. The variety of applications would not be limited by the availability of an injecting needle, necessitating visits to the doctor's office, and its use could be made more simple, more direct.

Soon after the initial synthesis of stilbestrol the first official notice of it appeared in a fifteen-paragraph article in the February 5, 1938, issue of the British magazine *Nature*.

The original stilbestrol was extremely potent, and Francis Dickens remembers that the powder was "very lightweight and flew around the laboratory. The British workmen making it inhaled some and later developed large breasts. They had problems putting their braces [suspenders] on." Dodds himself would later warn in a paper that men so exposed also experienced total impotence, and more than thirty years later an industrial accident in a Chicago chemical plant making DES injured numerous male workers.

Stilbestrol also had the advantage of being quite inexpensive. Susan Bell, a sociologist who wrote her 1980 doctoral dissertation at Brandeis University on DES, quoted government figures as showing that a gram of DES cost $2, while a gram of estradiol, a natural estrogen, cost $300. Robert H. Furman, M.D., the current medical director of Eli Lilly & Company, said in an interview that drug company costs were three hundred times more for a natural, injectable product than for DES.

The new compound was also not patented, a fact that apparently contributed to its widespread use in the United States. British custom at the time held that scientific work was done by scientists working for the public good and that such discoveries should be made available to the public without charge or cost. Michael B. Shimkin, a leading American cancer researcher, recalls visiting Dodds in 1939 or 1940 and learning of his anger at German scientists who were trying to corner the market on female sex hormones on behalf of the private German pharmaceutical combines.

"Dodds indicated to me that his main motivation [in being the first to synthesize a powerful, orally effective estrogen, which would stay in the public domain] was his anger at the patenting of molecules of estrogen by German firms," Shimkin said. In effect, Dodds wanted to produce something that the general public could get cheaply, without having to pay high prices to proprietary drug firms.

Dodds later went on to head the scientific committee of the British Empire Cancer Campaign and was a member of the American Association for Cancer Research. He was concerned from the very beginning about the cancer-causing potential of the new synthetic estrogen DES. Estrogens were known from animal and human studies to be carcinogenic. In one conversation with me Francis Dickens said, "There was concern all along about the cancer-causing potential of artificial sex hormones." Exactly how cancer was caused was an even greater mystery then than it is today, but people who know Dodds know he was concerned about it.

Because he was both a theoretician and a practicing medical man, Dodds also worried about the noncancerous effects of introducing any foreign substance into the infinitely complex female reproductive cycle. Several months after the original paper describing the synthesis of DES, Dodds and two colleagues published another paper (in the September 10, 1938, issue of the *British Medical Journal*), showing that DES administered by mouth to rats and rabbits would either prevent the implantation of the conceptus in the uterus or interrupt (and end) established pregnancies. It would, in fact, cause miscarriages in animals.

In the discussion section of the paper the authors stated: "Everything we know about the menstrual cycle of primates suggests that its hormonal control is the same as in lower animals, and it is extremely probable that the factors governing the implantation of the fertilized egg are fundamentally similar in women and lower animals. The experimental conclusions arrived at above should thus be applicable to women."

In effect, Dodds and his colleagues were setting out the theoretical basis for the "morning-after" pill, a controversial use to which DES was put in the 1960s. Dodds, however, according to his own writings and the recollections of his friends and colleagues, wanted no part in a morning-after pill or birth control pill, because he strongly felt that a woman's reproductive cycle was far too delicate a mechanism to bombard with exotic, powerful, foreign chemicals.

"Dodds always argued you should never have two unknowns," said Robert L. Noble, M.D., one of Dodds's coauthors on that paper. "Stilbestrol was an unknown, and the reproductive cycle was an unknown." Since their paper showed DES *caused* miscarriages, or prevented pregnancies in rabbits and rats, the idea of using DES to *prevent* miscarriages was nearly unthinkable to him, Noble said. "Nobody was using [DES] to prevent miscarriages except some crazy people in the United States. It was too radical a procedure," reported Noble, who is retired from his post as director of the Cancer Research Center at the University of British Columbia.

Within months of its 1938 synthesis, however, stilbestrol was being put to clinical tests in any circumstances in which female hormones were needed. In less than a year the Therapeutic Trials committee of the Medical Research Council in Great Britain reported favorably on the use of stilbestrol in amenorrhea (the absence or abnormal stoppage of the menstrual cycle), dysmenorrhea (painful menstruation), genital hypoplasia (incomplete development of the genitals), senile vaginitis (a thinning of the cells lining the vagina of postmenopausal women), and menopausal disorders. It was also used to suppress lactation in women who had just delivered babies. Tests from the United States, France, Germany, and Scandinavia were also favorable, although there was some concern in the U.S. about side effects, such as nausea.

In 1941, in America, J. A. Morrell, an E. R. Squibb & Sons medical researcher, published findings based on clinical reports on patients (unlike Dodds's early work, which had been based on laboratory studies on animals). In the *Journal of Clinical Endocrinology* he stated that more than 257 articles had already been written about DES, including many on its use for pregnant women. Among his conclusions: "No permanent toxic effects have been reported from liver function studies, blood or urine chemistry analyses or examinations of blood morphology and blood forming organs."

Another early use, one that is still in effect today, was developed in 1944 by University of Chicago cancer specialist Charles B. Huggins, who won the Nobel Prize in Physiology and Medicine for his use of DES in alleviating prostate cancer in men. The theory was classically simple: prostate cancer is caused in part by an increase in androgens. DES was used because, as a female sex hormone, it suppressed the production of androgens and the metabolism (or changes) of cells in the prostate. In its use in prostate cancer, DES became the world's first chemical to have any effect on any form of cancer when given by mouth. (Today there are some critics of this treatment who claim that stilbestrol use in such older patients is associated with an increase in heart problems.)

Dodds studied another use of DES in people during the 1940s and 1950s at Middlesex Hospital—the use of the drug on women with inoperable cancer of the breast. DES treatment was effective in lessening some pain and some growth of the cancerous lesions in only one out of five cases, he reported. But even Dodds, the man who had synthesized DES, was baffled as to why it should be effective. "It is very difficult to understand the action of stilbestrol in this condition, particularly when we consider that carcinoma of the breast can be produced in animals by its administration in certain circumstances," he wrote in a 1957 publication, *Biochemical Contributions to Endocrinology.*

The early clinical uses of DES mainly involved older, postmenopausal women. Dodds opposed the use of birth control pills precisely because so much was unknown about how the body functioned or how these powerful new chemicals would affect the body. H. G. Lazell, the retired chairman and chief executive officer of the British pharmaceutical company, the Beecham Group, told me during an interview in his London flat that Dodds, aware that DES caused breast cancer in test animals, single-handedly kept the firm from marketing a birth control pill, "because he was convinced that later in life women would get breast cancer."

For years Dodds was the chief medical consultant to Beecham's and sat in on all the board meetings. "He had a lively appreciation of the dangers of the hormone area," Mr. Lazell said. That appreciation extended to the use of DES as a growth stimulant in animals, a use he championed as long as the pellets of DES implanted in the neck or heads of animals were removed at least a week before slaughter, so that DES would not still be in the animal when its meat entered the food chain. DES stimulated animal growth by, in effect, forcing the body's cells and organs to grow faster. But regarding the use of DES by women during their reproductive years, Mr. Lazell added, "I don't think Charlie was very enthusiastic about the wide-spread use of stilbestrol, because of the same fears he had about the use of [any] hormones in pregnancy."

Sir Charles Dodds made his own comment about the early and enthusiastic use of his development. In a 1963 London lecture (printed two years later in "The Scientific Basis of Medicine: Annual Reviews: 1965,") he wrote:

> It is interesting to speculate in parenthesis on the differences in attitude toward new drugs thirty years ago and today. Within a few months of the first publication of the synthesis of stilbestrol, the substance was being marketed throughout the world. No long-term toxicity tests on animals such as dogs were ever done with stilbestrol and I suppose we have to be very thankful that it did prove to be such a non-toxic substance. When one considers the long series of tests that would be required, let us say by the American authorities, before the drug could be put on the market, it is really surprising that we escaped pharmacological disasters until a few years ago.

When Dodds was speaking, the thalidomide tragedy was fresh in the minds of people around the world, especially in England.

Sir Edward Charles Dodds, M.D., Ph.D., M.V.O., was an international scientific statesman. Honorary Fellow of the Royal College of Pathologists, the Royal College of Physicians and Surgeons (Canada), and an Australian Postgraduate Fellow in Medicine, he held honorary degrees from universities at Cambridge (England), Glasgow, Bologna, and Chicago. He delivered endowed lectures in Dublin, Stanford University (Palo Alto, California), and a dozen others. He was president of the 4th International Congress of Endocrinology in 1968; chairman of the Scientific Advisory Committee, British Empire Cancer Campaign; and chairman of the Science Committee of the British Heart Foundation. He was an honorary member of the American Society of Clinical Pathologists; the American Association for Cancer Research; the New York Academy of Sciences; the Biological Society of Chile; the Society of Chemical Industries of France; the Finnish Society of Medicine; the Royal Medical Academy of Barcelona; the Italian Chemical Society; the Danish Society of Internal Medicine; the Medical Society of Gothenburg (Sweden); and numerous others.

As a key transitional figure in the twentieth-century marriage of pure science and applied technology, he served with organizations in England dealing with food additives and poisonous substances in agricultural use. He was also an outside consultant, or informal adviser, to corporations around the world. Outside consultants are frequently asked by major corporations to bring them independent views and opinions unfettered by the fear of offending jealous bosses or protective administrators. Their use was first advocated by American firms, and subsequently the services of such independent specialists have been utilized by companies around the globe seeking to bring "American know-how" to their industries. Outside consultants are to some degree princes of the commercial world. They practice a type of scientific *noblesse oblige:* if they are asked their opinions, they give them; if they are not asked, so be it.

Dodds was a paid adviser to the Beecham Group in England. In the United States Dodds was a consultant to the giant American drug firm Carter-Wallace, Inc., the makers of the tranquilizer Miltown, among other products. According to Frank M. Berger, M.D., the retired president of Wallace Laboratories (the pharmaceutical division of the firm), Dodds "strongly disapproved of DES in contraceptive pills because of all the possible side effects."

Sir Ralph Dodds stood in front of the fireplace in his suburban London home and recalled that his father had also been a consultant to the Coca-Cola Company and the J. Walter Thompson advertising company, advising each through his expertise on food additives and public attitudes toward food consumption.

Sir Edward Charles Dodds had synthesized DES in 1938, and he kept a close watch on its use throughout the world. He lectured and wrote extensively on its actions, as far as they were understood. As late as 1962 the private Savage Club in London printed a cartoon of Dodds sitting at an upright piano, playing away, following the notes on sheet music clearly labeled "stilboestrol."

In view of the paper he coauthored in 1938 showing that DES caused miscarriages in pregnant rabbits and rats, his lifelong opposition to the use of birth control pills, and his extensive consulting work with major corporations and government agencies around the world, I was curious as to whether Dodds might have been a consultant to any of the companies that made DES for use in pregnancy.

A number of the people who knew him best, including his son, his secretary, and a leading American scientist, believe he was a consultant to Eli Lilly & Company, based in Indianapolis, Indiana, which was apparently the world's largest manufacturer of DES for all purposes, as well as the maker of hundreds of other drug products.

"Yes, he was a Lilly consultant—he went to the United States from the 1930s onward," his son said.

"Yes, he went to Indianapolis every nine months or so for years," Esme Barron recalled.

"Dodds was a consultant to Lilly," said Noble Laureate Charles B. Huggins. "He gave them cephalosporin, an antibiotic that cures certain bacterial diseases that Streptomyces [a natural source of antibiotics] won't touch. He thought it was wonderful." (Huggins added that he thought the association between DES and vaginal cancer was "a put-up job, the whole thing is nonsense, a legal gimmick to cheat Eli Lilly out of millions of dollars.")

Francis Dickens recalled: "Once in the late 1920s we went to an Oxford Street restaurant, a bunch of us scientists, and Dodds told us not to worry about the tab—we understood Eli Lilly would pay for it. I have a vague recollection [Dodds] was attached to them somehow. They supplied us with parathyroid glands from sheep. It was a very minor activity."

Eli Lilly & Company was a major American manufacturer of DES for use during pregnancy, for menopausal uses, and for use as a growth stimulant in animals. Two Lilly officials, the chief legal counsel, Raymond Rauch, and the chief medical officer, Robert H. Furman, M.D., said during an interview that to the best of their knowledge Dodds was not a Lilly consultant. Rauch said that the company "was aware" of Dodds's work and that he may have had some contact with Lilly through the head of its manufacturing plant in Basingstoke, England. A letter to me on December 21, 1981, from a Lilly public relations official stated, "Was Dr. E. C. Dodds a consultant to Lilly in the manufacturing of DES? No, he was not."

A globe-spanning corporation such as Eli Lilly, which currently has operations in sixty foreign countries, and had sales in 1980 of $2.5 billion (slightly more than the gross national product of Iceland), often works with outside consultants to gain the maximum possible knowledge about a product or drug compound. Company publications show that it worked with the Canadian developers of insulin in 1922 and with scientists working on cures for pernicious anemia, secondary anemia, and other medical problems. The company's reputation for innovative drug uses is widespread. H. G. Lazell of the Beecham Group said he held "Eli Lilly in high regard. They certainly had the trust of the medical profession."

Within the medical profession there was no one who knew more about DES than Sir Charles Dodds, whose friends remember him as fiercely proud of the product he had synthesized but who disapproved of the use of any foreign substances that might have an impact on the female reproductive system.

There may be no exact way of knowing whether Dodds was ever

asked his opinion of DES use during pregnancy, or, if he gave it, how it was received. Nowhere in any of his writings—even in the papers and lectures he gave through the 1960s, when DES was still experiencing widespread acceptance in the United States—is there any mention of the use of DES in pregnancy, much less his position on its use. Following his instructions, Esme Barron burned all Dodds's personal papers after his death. None of the people who say he was a Lilly consultant recalls his saying anything connecting his work for Lilly with its marketing of DES during pregnancy.

Dodds died in 1973, two years after American cancer specialists at Massachusetts General Hospital had linked the startling appearance of clear-cell adenocarcinoma in young girls with DES use by their mothers during pregnancy. "Those reports cut him up very badly," Sir Ralph Dodds remembers. "He would be very gloomy about it, he would say, 'We never designed it for that.' He would say, 'Of course, we never did the tests, for cancer of the prostate either, but it never worked out that way." But he was on record as firmly opposing the introduction of strong foreign chemicals into the healthy and functioning female body.

There is one final element in the Dodds story, one that if nothing else clearly shows his own attitude toward the proper use of the synthetic hormone he had shepherded into existence in 1938. Edward Charles Dodds was knighted in 1964 in recognition of his long career of service both to international medicine and to the British pharmaceutical companies he helped with guidance and advice.

When he was knighted he was eligible to have a stained glass window in his honor put up in the Hall of the Worshipful Society of Apothecaries of London, an ancient building off Blackfriars Lane, near the City of London, the historic financial center. To get there you follow a winding, cobblestoned street, keeping a sharp lookout for the small brass plaque on the wall announcing the Society. Walk up the impressive center staircase to the Great Hall, and in the far right-hand window, near the center, is Sir Edward Charles Dodds's heraldic crest.

John Brooke-Little, the Norroy and Ulster King of Arms—or senior herald of the Royal College of Arms—helped Dodds design the coat of arms. At the top is a woman in a blue off-the-shoulder dress holding an open book on which is written the chemical formula for diethylstilbestrol. The open book with the DES formula symbolized the fact that the compound had not been patented and was as available as an open book to anyone who wanted it. Mr. Brooke-Little explained that Dodds originally wanted the woman at the top of the coat of arms to be bare-breasted, because DES had been of use in alleviating inoperable breast cancer, but when his wife objected to the nudity he agreed to cover her up with the blue dress, a color his wife chose.

Beneath that is the knight's traditional helmet and mantling. Below that is the crest—two capons flanking a steer's head, to indicate the use of DES in animals. In the far left-hand corner is an upraised bloody hand, the traditional symbol for all baronets.

Beneath that a hand reaches downward from a symbolic cloud, the heraldic statement that in 1962 Dodds had served as president of the Royal College of Physicians. Beneath that two crabs are impaled by swords, meaning that cancer (symbolized by its astrologic sign, the crab) could be killed by the sword of DES.

Below that is Dodds's personal motto, Deeds Not Thoughts. The motto represents Dodds's own belief that science should produce products to benefit mankind rather than propose abstract concepts with no real-life application.

But nowhere on the coat of arms, designed by Dodds as his personal memorial, is there one hint of DES use in preventing miscarriages. Mr. Brooke-Little said the subject never came up.

4
DES ARRIVES IN THE UNITED STATES

It is almost as if, as DES crossed the Atlantic and passed through U.S. Customs, a change came over its use, background, and potential. American social and medical customs took over this potent new drug, marking it forever with a stamp as unique and distinctive as any stamp on a passport.

It is customary now to say, in a calming and reassuring way, that DES was used in pregnancy only between 1947, when the FDA approved its use for that purpose, and 1971, when approval for that purpose was withdrawn. But the fact is that just about one year after its synthesis in England, DES was being used during pregnancy in the United States.

Apparently the first doctor to use it in this way was an iconoclastic Houston gynecologist, Karl John Karnaky, M.D. "I got pure DES from Dodds, but I never met him," Karnaky said in a telephone interview. Acting as his intermediaries—in fact, the people who had suggested he use DES in the first place—were top executives of E. R. Squibb & Sons, later a major manufacturer of DES for pregnancy use. America and American medicine in those days were vastly different from what they are today. The country was made up of far more individualistic regions, and physicians operated with far more autonomy than is now the case. Karl John Karnaky was one of the first physicians who would help put Texas on the medical map. Karnaky, an unrepentant believer in

DES—the abbreviation he claims he devised—said that in his long career he has given it to more than 150,000 pregnant women.

Karnaky published the very first report regarding DES use during pregnancy to prevent spontaneous abortions. It appeared in the September 1942 issue of the *Southern Medical Journal*. The term "spontaneous abortion" was used in years past to identify what today would be called a miscarriage. In his report, which was widely read by other physicians and U.S. drug companies, Karnaky summarized DES work that had been going on at his clinic for the previous three years—since 1939.

Karnaky's great professional interests were and are menstrual disorders in general and the endometrium—the lining of the womb—in particular. Independently wealthy, he helped set up the Menstrual Disorder Clinic at Jefferson Davis Hospital in Houston, the first place in this country where DES was given to prevent miscarriages.

Karnaky's own work led him to believe that a withdrawal of estrogen was associated with cases of premature labor and threatened and habitual spontaneous abortions, although he acknowledged work done by Zondek, Aschheim, and Parkes (a coauthor of Dodds's) showing that estrogens caused abortions in animals.

In the 1942 *Southern Medical Journal* he described how the administration of DES in tablet form, and by injection in an oily solution into the anterior wall of the cervix, had worked. In 59 cases of inevitable spontaneous abortion, women arriving at his hospital with labor pains and some vaginal bleeding were injected with 25 to 100 milligrams of stilbestrol in oil. "Much to our surprise, after stilbestrol was given the labor pains stopped almost immediately or within 30 or 60 seconds, and did not recur for from 5 to 5½ hours. The stopping of labor pains by an estrogen is just the opposite of what we have been taught to expect." Another patient was mentioned, who had been given both injections of DES and DES tablets. "The pain of uterine cramping was gone in 45 seconds by the watch." The implication was clear in these few cases, he stated: stop the pain, and you stop the miscarriage.

Other patients he wrote about were also given DES, this time only in tablet form, with similar positive results reported. He went on to say: "The new synthetic estrogenic hormone, stilbestrol, can be used for the treatment of premature labor, threatened and habitual abortion . . . We can give too little stilbestrol but we cannot give too much." Consistent with good medical practice, he added, "Bed rest, thyroid, and vitamins should be given if indicated in these cases."

That last bit of advice—advocating bed rest along with DES—is, in hindsight, one of the little cracks in the façade of DES therapy that crops up repeatedly throughout the years. It is entirely possible to argue that bed rest, and not DES, was responsible for many successful pregnancies. The recommendation of bed rest in Karnaky's paper, however, shows that the notion was a constant companion of DES use right from the very start.

But Karnaky's conclusion was startling, and with it began the era of DES use during pregnancy in this country: "Stilbestrol can be used for the treatment of premature labor, threatened and habitual labor." Only sixty-eight years after Sir William Gull had laid down the principles of endocrinology, only nineteen years after Allen and Doisy had pinpointed the exact location of ovarian hormones, only four years after Sir Charles Dodds had synthesized the world's first synthetic estrogen, a way may have been found to fight the age-old problem of the woman's body that was unable or unwilling to carry a pregnancy to term.

It is customary at medical conferences, such as the one at which Karnaky delivered his paper, for other physicians with a similar interest to be called on for comment. Those comments are also published so that physicians reading the article can judge peer response to new findings. Willard M. Allen, M.D., from St. Louis, cautiously stated that he found the conclusions interesting, but added: "Of course, it would take a considerable period of time to determine whether the estrogen is truly beneficial in threatened abortion . . . The use of stilbestrol as shown by Dr. Karnaky is certainly as promising as any of the other methods of endocrine therapy which have been proposed, and in addition has the merit of being moderately inexpensive."

Frederick V. Emmert, M.D., also of St. Louis, said that treatment of threatened abortion with estrogenic injections had been tried fifteen years earlier (in the mid-1920s), but the results were not too encouraging. He also said:

I am astonished to learn that oral administration of massive doses of stilbestrol by Dr. Karnaky were well tolerated. This is in contrast with the observations of others that stilbestrol causes nausea and vomiting in non-pregnant cases . . . The high cost of potent progestin preparations [hormones also used to prevent miscarriages] prohibits their use in many instances. Medication with stilbestrol is very economical and thus benefits the masses. If Dr. Karnaky's deductions are confirmed by further investigations, his experiments will have opened up a new and promising field for therapeutic effort.

One physician was openly skeptical. William Bickers, M.D., from Richmond, Virginia, said Karnaky was operating on the assumption that threatened abortion was an "endocrine disease," when his own research indicated that it was more related to contractions in the uterus, which DES would not affect.

Four years later, in 1946, George V. S. Smith, M.D., Olive Watkins Smith, Ph.D., and others, would publish their own pro-DES paper. However, they criticized Karnaky's belief in the benefits of DES when injected into the cervix, claiming that the act of the injection itself might stimulate a nervous-system response that would stop the bleeding.

But all the elements were there in Karl John Karnaky's 1942 paper: the miraculous speed with which DES seemed to work (". . . the labor pains stopped almost immediately or within 30 to 60 seconds . . . the pain of uterine cramping was gone in 45 seconds by the watch . . ."); the concept that as an estrogen it somehow strengthened the ability of the pregnancy to survive; that it could be taken orally; that it was low in cost.

Karnaky's first knowledge of DES is significant for the light it sheds on the corporate interest in promoting the drug. As Karnaky said in an interview: "I was doing work in endometriosis and menstrual problems, and here come Dr. Sidney Newcomer and Dr. (J. A.) Morrell from E. R. Squibb and Co. [who] wanted to come to Houston and talk to me about something very valuable. They said, 'You seem to be the only one who's getting any articles published and doing any work on estrogens, and we have a synthetic one.' So they came to Houston, fed me and dined me . . . and I started using it."

In the custom of the day, Karnaky kept his own group of test animals, and he used dogs for experimental purposes. "I had this animal house, but the dang dogs were dying like flies. So I wrote Squibb and I said, 'Sidney, I don't want to work with this because it's killing all the dogs'—which we got for free from the dog pound across the street—but he said, 'No, no, I'll send you human experiment [doses] from Dodds.' And they sent me 0.1, 0.25, 1 milligram, 5 milligrams, and 25 milligrams of stilbestrol directly from England." Karnaky said it turned out that dogs were sensitive to DES, "but nothing else is. . . . You can treat any menstrual disorder with DES," he claimed.

E. C. Dodds had tested DES first on animals. Karl John Karnaky gave DES directly to pregnant patients. He reported his observations without comparing them to a control group (a group of people treated identically except that they weren't given the drug). He was acting along standard medical lines of his day, using the same methods other physicians were using.

At the same time Karnaky was giving DES to patients at his Menstrual Disorder Clinic in Houston other researchers around the country were giving DES to animals in an attempt to determine exactly how it worked and what the consequences might be. Mammary cancer in susceptible strains of mice after treatment with estrogens had been reported as early as 1932 by the French scientist A. Lacassagne. In 1939 Charles F. Geschickter, M.D., of Johns Hopkins University in Baltimore reported in *Radiology* that mammary cancer had been produced in rats by injecting them with DES as well as with other estrogens. He used Wistar rats in his experiments precisely because they did not have a history of spontaneously developing cancer.

In the October 1940 issue of the *Journal of the National Cancer Institute*, federal researchers Michael B. Shimkin and Hugh G. Grady wrote that DES produced breast cancers in both male and female mice. In the strain used, C3H mice, the females had been deliberately bred to spontaneously produce breast cancer, but the male mice did not normally develop it. The presence of breast cancer in male mice was a testament to the potency of DES. Shimkin, who later was medical director of the National Cancer Institute, had gotten the DES directly from Charles Dodds.

In 1939 and 1940 Northwestern University Medical School faculty members R. R. Greene, M. W. Burrill, and A. C. Ivy published a number of articles in scientific journals, such as the *American Journal of Anatomy* and *Science*, on the subject "Experimental Intersexuality," showing the impact on animal fetuses when the pregnant mothers had been treated with estrogens, including DES. Female rat offspring had enlarged uteruses and structural changes in the vagina and ovaries. Male rat offspring had small and improperly developed penises and changes in other male sexual and reproductive systems. Forty years later, with hindsight, their work would be seen as being predictive of changes that women and men exposed *in utero* to DES might experience. In one of their articles, however, the authors pointed out that it wasn't clear why these changes had occurred and bent over backward to state that the changes might be "apparent and not real." But they never suggested their findings were false or due to chance, and they never backed away from them.

In the April 1941 issue of *Endocrinology*, H. O. Burdick and Helen Vedder from Alfred University, in upstate New York, published an article showing why Dodds and his coworkers had been able to interrupt pregnancies in rats and rabbits. DES, they showed, caused the ova (female eggs) to "disintegrate after both large and small doses of stilbestrol."

Also in April 1941, Yale University researchers Edgar Allen, Ph.D., and W. U. Gardner, Ph.D., published an article in *Cancer Research* on the general ability of estrogens to cause cervical cancer in animals. They concluded: "The high incidence of cervical cancer in these experimental groups emphasizes that estrogen is a very important factor, not merely an incidental one, in cervical carcinogenesis." But they also made this interesting point: "One reason why the incidence of cancer of the cervix uteri has been so low in mice treated with estrogens is that mammary cancer appears at an earlier age than does cervical cancer, and consequently animals may die of the former; *i.e.*, many of them do not live long enough for the cervical cancer to develop."

In short, precise animal studies such as these were going on at a number of major research centers around the country showing the ability of DES to cause cancer and also somehow interfere with the normal development of the sexual and reproductive systems of offspring born to pregnant animals treated with DES.

At the same time, however, two famous Boston endocrinologists believed that DES might help them in their goal of helping women have babies.

5

CONFLICTING REPORTS
SHOWING THAT DES
PREVENTED
MISCARRIAGES—OR DIDN'T

Their rambling old house in the Brookline section of Boston is, they say, a national monument, and it is likely that if it hadn't been for DES, they incontrovertibly would be too.

George Van Siclen Smith, M.D., and Olive Watkins Smith, Ph.D., were for years professionally regarded as the first couple in endocrinology. Both were Harvard-trained; in 1929 she was the first woman to receive a Ph.D. degree from Harvard's graduate school of medical science. He headed Harvard's gynecology department from 1942 to 1967.

In the course of their long and distinguished careers they separately or jointly published more than 260 medical papers—10 of his were published while he was still a *medical student*—in the fields of endocrinology and cancer research. Raising their own colony of animals in order to ensure the uniform response of the animal host—a widely accepted concept today that almost no one else was following then—they were the first, or among the first, to show that diabetics need more insulin during pregnancy than do nondiabetics. They were also the first to obtain estradiol, the potent naturally occurring estrogen, from humans. And they worked out the biosynthetic process of estrogen metabolism years before other researchers fully appreciated the value of their work.

They are also the two best known medical advocates of the use of DES during pregnancy to prevent miscarriages, and the consequences of that now haunt their old age.

The presence of adenosis does not worry them, "because there has yet to be a case of adenosis going on to cancer," Olive W. Smith said when I spoke with them in the large old-fashioned kitchen in their home. Now in her eighties, Olive Smith speaks sharply, with precision, often acting as the spokesman for both, whose careers were linked for so long. The existence of structural and anatomic changes in the reproductive tracts of DES daughters may exist, she said, because they are the daughters of women with similar problems. "But we would like to have before we die assurance that cancer had nothing to do" with DES use.

The Smiths were important transitional figures on the medical scene. Before World War II, gynecologists just treated the existing pregnancy; they never measured the biochemical changes a pregnant woman was going through, in part because the tools didn't exist. George Smith, a gynecologist, and Olive Smith, an endocrinologist, were in the first generation of American scientists to try to measure what was happening inside the human body. George Smith is also praised by his colleagues as much for his surgical technique as for his frequent advice to women to *avoid* surgery. He held an endowed chair at Harvard, but his annual earnings in 1942 were only $2,500—a figure that if computed at a 1982 rate would bring him only $20,250 annually. By contrast, other men of his stature today receive upward of $100,000 annually in salary.

The work of the Smiths in the 1930s involved trying to discover why pregnancies failed—in medical language, what the toxemias of pregnancy were. This led them to develop their own animal colonies, to work with insulin for diabetic mothers, to seek out precisely the ways in which the body's chemistry changed and reacted during pregnancy. "It's the sort of work you can spend years on and nobody will understand," Olive Smith said reflectively.

George Smith was a teacher and a university researcher who treated patients in his small private practice. As both a university scientist and a physician who was especially concerned about pregnant women, he understood at close range the agony and trauma of women who miscarried. He saw the faces of the women—one out of five—who lost their babies.

And that was their purpose. "We wanted to save babies!" George

Smith said strongly. "We read Dodds's paper on stilbestrol [in 1938]," Olive Smith added. "We said it's estrogenic, cheap, oral, we ought to be studying patients. We wrote to Dr. Newcomer at Squibb for a supply of stilbestrol. He sent us a bottle in crystalline form. We put it into capsules." Because George Smith was a gynecologist, and did not himself treat pregnant women, the Smiths gave the DES they had prepared to obstetricians, who gave it to their patients, and then the Smiths measured the biochemical results.

Their theory was simple and logical, and because of their reputations and the results they reported, it became widely accepted in the American medical community: progesterone, a hormone that helps prepare the uterus to receive and maintain a fertilized egg, is needed for a successful pregnancy. The secretion of progesterone, they felt, could be stimulated by DES, which produced all the regular actions of estrogens. But since it was then impossible to measure the level of progesterone in a woman's body, they sought to measure pregnanediol, which is produced by progesterone. Pregnanediol appears in the urine. If there was more pregnanediol, there must be more progesterone, Olive Smith reasoned. So when DES was given, pregnanediol was measured, using a new technique called the Venning method: a pregnant woman's urine was crystallized, then the resulting crystals were separated and weighed. Using this technique, they determined that pregnanediol increased as DES was given. The Venning method was not only the latest tool in the field, it was virtually the only tool for sensitive measurements of this kind.

Progesterone itself, the hormone everyone was after, was available then only in highly expensive natural form, costing at least a hundred fifty to three hundred times more than DES. And it had to be administered by injection, a discomforting process in itself and one that required the patient to come to the doctor's office. That is why DES seemed to the Smiths to be such an important chemical.

The results that the Smiths obtained, first with another researcher named Priscilla White and then by themselves, were startling and encouraging: women given DES did seem to be having an increase in pregnanediol, and they were also having more babies, despite many previous miscarriages.

In 1946 the Smiths and David Hurwitz, M.D., coauthored an article in the *American Journal of Obstetrics and Gynecology*. Their conclusions, backed up by meticulous detail, were impressive. Nearly every sentence was cross-referenced to an earlier study the Smiths had done on a technical aspect of the theory, and they explained their thought processes simply and clearly: DES could be used to prevent miscarriages in certain women, mainly those who had had miscarriages previously.

The theory was based on the Smiths's work with pregnant women, including pregnant diabetic women, who lacked normal progesterone secretion late in their troubled pregnancies. To test the scientific theory that DES could be used to stimulate the production of progesterone, the Smiths and Hurwitz gave the example of one woman, "Mrs. M.K., aged 36 years, gravida iii [third pregnancy]." She had had a stillborn child in 1934 and a living child born with pregnancy complications in 1938. In 1944, when referred to Hurwitz and analyzed by the Smiths, she was pregnant, diagnosed as diabetic, and weighed 210 pounds. She was given DES pills in her seventeenth week of pregnancy, and continued taking them almost continuously until the thirty-fifth week. She delivered an 8-pound baby without complications.

The paper stated: "The urinary excretions of pregnanediol rose steadily while diethylstilbestrol was being taken, and dropped precipitously each time it was omitted. . . . [This] provides fairly conclusive evidence that diethylstilbestrol was responsible for the steady rise in pregnanediol excretion, presumably as a result of the progesterone stimulation." The title to the short, five-page article stressed the use of DES "with special reference to the prevention of late pregnancy accidents." But in the text of the piece the authors stated: "The progesterone stimulating properties of diethylstilbestrol make it an equally logical agent for the prevention of accidents in early pregnancy."

Late pregnancy accidents, early pregnancy accidents—the seeds were being sown for DES use in all pregnancy accidents, for the prevention of pregnancy accidents.

Over the years the Smiths's theory has been criticized as being wrong, with some researchers even today claiming that they had measured the wrong chemical substances. The Smiths have always denied this, and in the late 1940s and early 1950s they and others produced additional papers backing up their original statements. And, significantly, no tests using today's more sophisticated techniques have ever been done in an attempt to prove them wrong. In an interview for this book, one world-renowned authority said that after studying the dispute he concluded that in fact the Smiths's theory was right.

In the summary to the 1946 article the authors added: "A regime of stilbestrol administration by mouth is proposed as a preventive measure to be tried in cases with a history of repeated accidents in pregnancy, which may be referable to progesterone deficiency, namely, abortion, premature delivery, pre-eclampsia [a pregnancy condition associated with hypertension, among other things], or intrauterine death."

Advocating a gradual increase of DES in 5-milligram doses, the authors asked readers to send them their case reports if they used this therapy.

The authors pointed out in the 1946 paper that DES was being given because of its ability to stimulate progesterone, and nowhere in the paper was there a reference to the known potency of DES as an estrogen.

In retrospect, that may have turned out to be too fine a scientific point to apply to so new a chemical; whether DES stimulated progesterone or not, easily available animal studies showed it was potent. By concentrating on the progesterone-stimulating ability of DES, the Smiths were possibly conditioning themselves, and almost certainly others, to ignore the studies showing it caused cancer and anatomical abnormalities in animals. By concentrating on the possible benefits and ignoring the possible harm, they were very much a part of the medical establishment and temper of their times.

Ignoring the possible risks, or side effects, of a substance was and is a common social and scientific procedure. In the industrial world, toxic wastes are buried precisely because they are toxic. The fact that they are sufficiently potent to cause harm years after their disposal is an unintended side effect. The contemporary chemical world is aware of Vietnam veterans who walked through areas once sprayed with Agent Orange and have reported horrible side effects on them and their children; American military techniques harming American soldiers is an unintended side effect.

The Smiths developed their theory in an age in which the emphasis was on the benefits, not on the risks. They always acted responsibly. The Smiths said they felt that by recommending limited doses they would avoid unintended side effects. That is why the agonizingly slow revelations of the impact of DES have created around George and Olive Smith the atmosphere almost of a contemporary tragedy: the clash between two inevitable forces, the desire to prevent miscarriages and the potential danger of the drug that seemed able to prevent them.

In short, there was enough in the 1946 article for anyone to come away with something: it was recommended by the Smiths of Harvard for accidents of late pregnancy, early pregnancy, repeated accidents of pregnancy, abortion, and premature delivery. And it was capped with the statement that the DES therapy "is proposed as a preventive measure to be tried" when problems seemed to be arising.

Looking back at that time in medical history, Ann B. Barnes, M.D. (a coprincipal investigator of the federally funded DESAD project, which has sought to measure the impact of DES exposure on mothers and their offspring), said, "DES was naively given into the black box [of the human body] with a lack of understanding of the complexities involved. So was progesterone, so was alcohol. It was the beginning of the era of wanting to do things for people, but a lot of obstetricians in those days were male midwives. Half of all deliveries were by general practioners, GPs," she said.

In the 1940s there were 179,856 medical doctors in the United States, but in 1945 there were only 1,960 gynecologists certified by the American Board of Obstetrics and Gynecology, or slightly more than 1 percent. In the 1950s there were 219,997 medical doctors, but only 4,625 board-certified obstetrician-gynecologists, or 2 percent of the total. In the 1960s there were 260,484 M.D.s, and 8,283 board-certified Ob-Gyn's, or 3 percent of the total.

Even if one assumes, as is reasonable, that there were trained Ob-Gyn's who were not board-certified, and that there were therefore double the number given for that specialty, the figures still represent only 2, 4, and 6 percent respectively of specialists during the years of DES's greatest use.

Most doctors were general practitioners—GPs—and minutely documented reports coming from the most famous couple in endocrinology—coming from Harvard—and published in the *American Journal of Obstetrics and Gynecology* must have carried considerable weight.

A doctor doing nothing but seeing patients during office hours and working on hospital rounds might not have read Dodds's 1938 article showing DES caused miscarriages in rabbits; might not have read the Shimkin, Gestickter articles showing DES caused cancer in test animals; might not have read the Greene, Burrill, and Ivy studies, published in the *American Journal of Anatomy*, showing that DES caused structural abnormalities in the reproductive tracts of animals whose mothers received DES during pregnancy.

As we shall see, there were warnings against the use of estrogens published in the editorial sections of the *Journal of the American Medical Association* in 1939 and 1940, six years earlier. But if a physician recalled them, he might reasonably think that times and knowledge change.

DES was also a legal drug, approved in 1941 by a government

watchdog agency, the FDA, for use in various menopausal problems. Once it was initially approved, it could be used by physicians for any other purpose they deemed fit. In 1947 the FDA approved its use in pregnancy, and it was manufactured and marketed by companies with excellent reputations—Lilly, Squibb, Merck, Abbott.

It was baby-boom time, and the Smiths's theory seemed to make sense: DES stimulated progesterone, a fact that could be measured by pregnanediol. Increase progesterone and you help ensure a healthy pregnancy. The Smiths prescribed DES, claimed that their measurements showed an increase in pregnanediol, and then said that the women who had taken DES had more healthy children than women who had not taken DES.

But in less than a year their theory was challenged, and to some, demolished, by two physicians from the University of Chicago.

There are schools of thought in medicine, just as there are schools of thought in philosophy, economics, literary criticism, and wine tasting. Competition between rival schools is not restricted just to football teams in October. By what standards should something be judged? When should action be taken? When should it not be taken? What is the trade-off between potential benefit and potential risk?

In obstetrics the two schools of thought break down roughly along these lines: on one side is the school holding that pregnancy is too complicated and delicate a time for any intervention at all, regardless of the intention; on the other side is the school holding that under proper circumstances, with proper caution, intervention is acceptable.

It is impossible to say that these philosophical beliefs were held in only one part of the country or another, because various people in various parts of the country have expressed themselves on both sides of the issue. But generally speaking, the more activist philosophy, based on the latest techniques and findings, was based in the East, and the more hands-off philosophy was more midwestern.

M. Edward Davis, M.D., held a faculty appointment in the Department of Obstetrics and Gynecology at the University of Chicago. In 1940, in the *American Journal of Obstetrics and Gynecology*, he published a paper called simply "A Clinical Study of Stilbestrol." In this sixteen-page paper Davis described giving DES to terminally ill women and to women with various menopausal problems. His conclusions were encouraging. DES "has tremendous clinical possibilities . . . It replaces the estrogenic action of the ovary," he found, with action that he had earlier in the paper described as coming so fast that "many women expressed amazement at the result."

Davis was an advocate of estrogens; he thought they might be used almost forever. But in his paper he was extremely cautious: "The widespread clinical use of stilbestrol must await more adequate evidence as to its possible toxicity . . . Careful clinical observations must be continued with the most guarded approach until such time as the lack of toxicity of the drug can be firmly established." He did *not* use the drug during pregnancy, and he advised caution until more testing could be done.

In 1946 the Smiths published their famous paper, also in the *American Journal of Obstetrics and Gynecology*. The Smiths *did* recommend that the drug be given to pregnant women, and their correspondents around the country gave it to them, basing their action on a concept that *should* have worked: DES stimulated the production of progesterone, as measured by the increase in pregnanediol.

But Davis didn't believe it. Instead, he and Nicholas W. Fugo, a faculty member of the University of Chicago's Pharmacology Department, tested the Smiths's theory on a group of pregnant women, using their own techniques. If the Smiths were right, the level of pregnanediol, as measured by excreted urine, should increase after DES use.

It didn't, at least not when given early in pregnancy, which the Smiths had recommended for early pregnancy problems. "Diethylstilbestrol . . . when administered daily in large amounts over long periods during the first 16 weeks of gestation did not alter the normal excretion of pregnanediol . . . If it is desirable to increase the amount of progestational hormone available during early pregnancy, it is more logical to administer progesterone in liberal amounts rather than diethylstilbestrol," Davis and Fugo stated.

This refutation of the Smiths's work appeared in the *Proceedings of the Society for Experimental Biology and Medicine*, which is not widely read by street-level gynecologists, as is the *American Journal of Obstetrics and Gynecology*. Both studies had received DES from Squibb. Davis and Fugo made reference in their paper to the studies by Greene, Burrill, and Ivy, which had showed anatomical changes in animals after *in utero* DES treatment. But the Smiths, who had sixteen footnoted references, including ten to their own work, did not mention the earlier negative studies. They said during our interview that they felt careful, controlled dosages would avoid the problems animal researchers had encountered.

The Smiths disputed Davis and Fugo's findings then, and do so now, saying each study used different techniques, which ensured different results. The conflicting findings might have raised some questions in the minds of people disposed to be skeptical, but apparently they did not. Even if the Smiths's theory was right, it still ignored the dangers of estrogens.

The year 1947 was not a particularly good one for the pro-DES faction of the medical community, although, in retrospect, nothing seemed to slow them down. The twenty-fourth edition of the *Dispensatory of the United States of America*, an encyclopedia of medical and pharmacological information, was published, with this anti-DES zinger on page 363: "To date no national catastrophy [*sic*] has been recognized, but it is perhaps too early for any deleterious effect on the incidence of carcinoma of the female generative tract or breast to appear."

In November of 1947 Los Angeles physicians Gordon Rosenblum and Eugene Melinkoff published in the *Western Journal of Surgery* a generally favorable survey of DES literature, concluding with four thoughtful questions about potential dangers of DES. Stating that "it seems to us that its use is rational," they nevertheless wondered whether DES in large doses would cause pituitary or other glandular imbalance that would become evident later in life; whether DES in large doses was carcinogenic in people; whether DES would affect the glandular balance of the child *in utero*; and whether DES would give better results for the treatment of threatened or habitual miscarriages than other drugs.

Like Karl John Karnaky, when they administered DES they also advised patients in their study to get plenty of bed rest—the time-honored recommendation for pregnant women with a history of miscarriage. "At the onset of symptoms of threatened abortion the patient was ordered to bed and given per mouth 5 to 25 mg. of diethylstilbestrol at the first dose . . . so long as symptoms [of abortion] existed 25 mg. every hour was given so that some patients received as much as 200 mg. within 24 hours," they wrote. Regarding published reports of nausea and vomiting associated with DES use, the authors stated: "On the contrary many patients reported a feeling of well-being and lessening of nausea and headache after beginning the drug."

They were also in bed at the time.

The authors concluded by saying that "only time will tell" whether DES was the best endocrine solution to pregnancy loss. In the meantime, due to the low cost of DES compared to the high cost of progesterone, they said they liked to think of DES as the "Poor Woman's Progesterone."

In 1948 Olive Smith published another paper, also in the *American Journal of Obstetrics and Gynecology*, analyzing the results of 632 pregnancies handled by 117 obstetricians from Boston to Oakland. The results were also favorable to DES use. Women who were chronic aborters, she wrote, "were given small doses of stilbestrol during the cycle of conception . . . thereby providing a more normal maternal environment from the very start." Although Olive Smith indicated that the theory was aimed at women with a history of pregnancy complications, the language of the paper shows why it was so easy for physicians who were so inclined to start using DES for anything involving pregnancy, and why it was so easy for drug companies to keep manufacturing the drug and pushing it for all types of pregnancy problems of women who had miscarried before. The history of DES use in this country shows that that is precisely what happened.

Significantly, Olive Smith again stated with precision the hair-splitting concept that seems to have led to so many problems: "An important part of the understanding of this concept is the realization that stilbestrol is given not because it is estrogenic but because it stimulates the secretion of estrogen and progesterone."

DES did not enter the human body only as an estrogen-stimulating drug, however; it also entered it as an estrogen, with enormous, and unrealized, power.

Olive Smith warned against the overdosage of DES, but by and large the Smiths's analysis of studies done according to their plan was favorable.

In the spring of 1949 the Smiths traveled down to the Shenandoah Mountains to a resort in Hot Springs, Virginia, where they read a paper at the seventy-second annual meeting of the American Gynecological Society (the paper was later published in the *American Journal of Obstetrics and Gynecology*). They described their paper as "a report of continued progress" in the use of DES during the pregnancies of women with prior miscarriages, based on a two-year study from 1947 to 1949 at the Boston Lying-In Hospital. The results were the same as before: DES worked. And this time they compared the pregnancy experience of DES mothers with that of mothers who were not given DES.

Regarding premature births, they wrote: "DES [seemed to stimulate] better placental function and hence bigger and healthier babies by the time premature delivery occurred." As in all their studies, the Smiths were following standard practice in many medical studies—simply comparing their study group with another random group of people. So that reading this, a physician who had not followed the DES debate in the professional journals might think that all babies were bigger and healthier with DES use *in utero.*

This time, however, the air during the discussion period after the meeting was riddled with conceptual bullets aimed at their work. Their theory had previously been attacked by Davis and Fugo, who claimed that DES did not stimulate progesterone. Now their conclusions about the reason healthy babies were born to women given DES were also challenged. Ernest W. Page, M.D., of San Francisco wondered whether "unconscious factors of selection" could account for the threefold improved delivery rate when DES was used. Willard Allen, M.D., the early cautionary, asked whether DES might actually work to help the uterus physically relax, so that it could better accommodate the fetus, rather than have an effect through chemical means alone.

Most prophetically, William J. Dieckmann, M.D., from the University of Chicago, was openly skeptical: "Their results, presumably due to the administration of stilbestrol, are better than we have been able to accomplish by extensive and expensive prenatal care. I do not know what it is due to." And then Dieckmann made a statement showing how far medical techniques had developed in just a few short years. He pointed out that more than good medical care and concern were needed. Objective criteria and cold analysis were needed too, so he said: "I gather that the essayists have not used a placebo, which I think is important."

Dieckmann was a midwesterner, born in Belleville, Illinois, just before the turn of the century, so he was a contemporary of George Smith's, but one who differed with him in philosophy, and certainly on DES. Dieckmann was the associate editor of the *American Journal of Obstetrics and Gynecology,* in which so many of the Smiths's papers had appeared. A few years later, after he had seemingly demolished the Smiths's recommendation for DES, he would found the Society of Gynecologic Investigations.

Placebos (sugar pills, or pills with no active ingredients in them) were gaining wide acceptance as a control necessary to eliminate all psychological bias on the part of the examining doctor and on the part of the patient. For example, a woman using a drug might take better care of herself *in order to help the drug do its work* than a woman who was getting no drug at all.

To eliminate that possibility, Dieckmann was implying, everyone should get a pill—either DES or a sugar pill—so that treatment would be identical, *except for the use of the drug by some patients.* In the current Smith study one group of women had been given DES, but the other group had been given nothing at all.

In coming years the placebo procedure would be refined and modified into double-blind placebo-controlled studies in which even the examining doctors would not know which patient got what. In this way pure results, free of bias, could be obtained.

Dieckmann concluded by saying that as soon as one of his own projects was finished, he would adopt this plan to test the Smiths's conclusion. And he was not the only one. All over the country, physicians curious about the Smiths's remarkable results tried to duplicate them, using the latest intellectually progressive controlled studies rather than the services of a kindly assistant whom the Smiths had asked to do follow-up studies for them.

In 1950 three Navy medical officers, R. E. Crowder, E. S. Bills, and J. S. Broadbent, published (in the *American Journal of Obstetrics and Gynecology*) their own controlled study of one hundred pregnant women, showing that DES was no more effective in preventing miscarriages than bed rest and sedation alone. They made reference to the Davis and Fugo article, which had refuted the Smiths's chemical theory. "If stilbestrol does not stimulate the increased production of progesterone, its use in threatened abortion has no theoretical basis. The results of our study indicate that stilbestrol did not increase the number of pregnancies salvaged. We have therefore concluded that stilbestrol is of no value in the treatment of threatened abortion," they wrote.

It is significant also that they dealt with cases of threatened abortion (or miscarriage) in general and did not limit themselves only to women with prior histories of miscarriages. In effect, they were the first to test the Smiths's theory in the way the drug was being prescribed in the real world—to women with signs of miscarriage, whether or not they had previously had a miscarriage.

In 1952 the *American Journal of Obstetrics and Gynecology* punched another hole in the DES balloon, with an article using aggressively hostile language. Gynecologists David Robinson and Landrum B. Shettles stated:

> The synthetic estrogen, diethylstilbestrol, has more recently become a popular form of therapy in threatened abortion. The public has been so

frequently told of the virtue of this drug through articles appearing in lay journals that it now requires a courageous physician to refuse this medication. The mass of pharmaceutical literature, extolling the wonders of this drug, has also rendered practitioners amenable to his patient's demands. This situation, together with the understandable desire to do something positive toward rescuing a teetering pregnancy, has resulted in widespread use of diethylstilbestrol in threatened abortion.

Regarding miscarriages, Robinson and Shettles wrote that it is "not a single disease entity. It is an expression of multiple etiological agents," including defective eggs, X-ray therapy, trauma, anesthesia, vitamin deficiency, and anatomical abnormalities.

Regarding DES used in their controlled study of ninety-three pregnant women, they wrote, "These results give no evidence of a favorable therapeutic effect from diethylstilbestrol in threatened abortion . . . [DES] is, in fact, a dismal failure in the general treatment of threatened abortion."

In 1953, also in the *American Journal of Obstetrics and Gynecology,* James Henry Ferguson, M.D., wrote that he and his staff at Charity Hospital, in New Orleans, followed the Smiths's own prescribed regimen of DES in a controlled study of 184 women given DES, and 198 women given a placebo. His conclusion: "The stilbestrol has no effect . . ."

There are two interesting points to this study. One is that Ferguson directly refuted the Smiths's claims that premature babies whose mothers had been given DES were healthier: he found no significant difference. The second is that following the presentation of Ferguson's paper, a physician named R. R. Greene spoke up. Greene had coauthored the papers more than a decade earlier showing that DES caused structural abnormalities in animals born to mothers injected with it. If controls had been used in their early studies by the Smiths, he said, "there would probably be less glowing claims for stilbestrol as a universal panacea . . . Dr. Ferguson has, I believe, driven a very large nail into the coffin that we will use some day to bury some of the extremely outsized claims" for DES.

Eight months later, in November 1953, in the *American Journal of Obstetrics and Gynecology,* another large nail was driven into the DES coffin. William J. Dieckmann and three of his colleagues published not only a controlled study of DES use but a study that was double-blind as well. This is a controversial study, not in its precise medical techniques but in allegations about its ethics, because some of the women who went to the Chicago Lying-In Hospital for treatment claim they were never told they were being given DES, or were never told what the possible side effects might be.

UCLA professor Nicholas S. Assali, M.D., said in an interview that during the 1950s he visited his friend Dieckmann in Chicago and saw Dieckmann or an associate literally standing "at the door of the Lying-In Hospital to separate the patients into two groups," the group that would get DES and the group that would get the placebo. "I told him, 'Bill, this looks like Auschwitz or Buchenwald—this one goes to the gas chamber, this one goes to the crematorium. My gosh, you can't do a study like that.' "

Assali believes that the Smiths's theory was correct, though "by today's standards their methodology was primitive. But maybe twenty years from now our methodology will be seen as primitive too." He also believes that the Dieckmann study "didn't prove anything, because it used a variety of patients with a variety of problems." Assali has produced precise papers showing the influence of DES on pregnant sheep. But as Ann Barnes, M.D., pithily remarked, "A sheep ain't a person."

However, when the Dieckmann paper was first presented, with the Smiths in the audience, its conclusions were loud and clear, and they have never been refuted. It was the largest study yet (840 patients given DES following the Smiths's recommendations, 804 patients given an identical placebo) under controlled conditions of DES use in pregnancy, and it showed that DES "did not reduce the incidence of abortion, prematurity, or postmaturity. Premature babies . . . were no longer nor more mature for their gestational ages" (as the Smiths had claimed they would be) than babies of mothers who had taken the placebos. DES "did not decrease the incidence of prenatal mortality. It did not decrease the frequency of the toxemias of pregnancy."

George Smith defended their work before the audience at the Lake Placid, New York, hotel where the paper was read. Dieckmann had studied too many pregnant women with too many variations in their pregnancy histories. "We now wish they had run their experiment on normal primigravidas [women pregnant for the first time], thereby making it comparable to ours . . . We also wish we had given a placebo to our controls," he conceded, although he suggested that was a minor point. "Our experience with the use of stilbestrol continues to be satisfactory and to confirm our previously reported clinical results . . . We trust that the many obstetricians who have been following our recommendations for the use of stilbestrol in pregnancy will realize that the paper presented this morning and the report by Dr. Ferguson fail to provide definite evidence to the contrary."

Olive Smith added, "We have never said that it should be given to all women during pregnancy," but, she said, only to some for prevention of abortions. "It is not a panacea but only a therapeutic agent for the rational use of which there exists a sound rationale."

Brian Little, M.D., from Boston, supported the Smiths and said: "I think the Chicago group has misinterpreted the Smiths . . . Dr. Dieckmann has chosen all 2,000 clinic patients, including women [having first, second, or third child, and women in various medical conditions], whereas the Smiths chose a specific group, the primigravidas . . . the figures that are reported in each paper cannot be compared for they do not represent the same entities." Based on his own work, Little stated, "stilbestrol and other endocrine therapy should be used in diabetes and habitual aborters, at least. Recognizing that it is premature to make any startling conclusions, many of us feel that this treatment is certainly on the right track."

Willard Allen, M.D., the ongoing skeptic, now spoke up again, echoing a view widely held at the time.

> Many practicing physicians have come to believe that stilbestrol is a panacea. . . . It would seem to me, therefore, that these results indicate that stilbestrol for routine use has little value . . . It seems to me that little more is to be gained by future studies of this sort. Further studies should be directed to the study of stilbestrol or other hormones in patients whose past obstetrical performance indicates a good likelihood of recurring trouble or in cases where difficulty with the particular pregnancy has already occurred.

M. Edward Davis made the closing remarks. He had been the co-author of the article in 1947 that challenged the very biochemical basis on which the Smiths were using DES. He was also one of Dieckmann's coauthors on this study. "We have followed Dr. Olive Smith's work very carefully. This experiment was designed in an attempt to learn whether diethylstilbestrol has therapeutic value. We have not proved that it is of value . . . it will take at least as many more patients just as carefully controlled to prove that stilbestrol administered prophylactically to normal or abnormal pregnant patients has any value . . ."

Those studies have never been made.

George and Olive Smith were functioning as part of a system that wanted to prevent miscarriages, that was looking for a tool to accomplish its purpose. And when that tool was found they happily gave it to women who had *also* been looking for it. The Smiths had been dealing with a small number of women with certain medical problems, but very quickly their theory was, without testing, applied to any woman in any state of pregnancy. Doctors were willing to overlook the potential dangers when faced with patients they wanted to help, patients who asked for—and sometimes demanded—help.

But it is also true that once the large, broadly based critical studies had been made, no one, especially the drug companies, ever retested the drug under the more limited conditions that the Smiths to this day say would be appropriate.

As the 1950s were coming to a close, it might be thought that at least doctors who had somehow missed the debates raging like mud fights in the professional journals might be excused for not being aware of the doubts and disagreements. Except that if they were in medical school at the time, a standard textbook also had a few choice words to say about DES. Called *The Pharmacological Basis of Therapeutics*, it was written by Louis S. Goodman, M.D., from the University of Utah, and Alfred Gilman, Ph.D., from the Albert Einstein College of Medicine, at Yeshiva University, in New York. Two different disciplines—one medical, one scientific—and two different geographical locations—one the Far West, one the east coast—combined in their backgrounds. The book is regarded as the bible in its field.

On the subject of estrogens in pregnancy they wrote: "Studies of the pharmacological actions of estrogens in animals have shown that they [estrogens] are capable of producing abortions. Therefore, it required temerity on the part of obstetricians to use estrogens [in pregnancy]. In the opinion of many, the value of estrogens in these conditions is still unproved."

The authors described the work of the Smiths, saying it was on that basis that DES was used in pregnancy, but noted that the Smiths's claim that DES chemically stimulated progesterone production had been challenged by Davis and Fugo, among others. In addition, the clinical results achieved by the Smiths, ostensibly demonstrating that DES reduced miscarriages, were also challenged by Dieckmann, among others. Goodman and Gilman further said that estrogens are "well tolerated" during pregnancy, but the claim that they "reduce the incidence of abortion or favorably affect the complications of pregnancy is based upon reports which require confirmation by scrupulously controlled studies . . . Certainly the available evidence does not justify the routine use of estrogens" in pregnancy.

So now everyone, young doctors as well as old, could have been up-to-date. The Dieckmann study came out in 1953, the textbook in 1958. For nearly *two decades* after the Dieckmann study, DES stayed on the shelves of American pharmacies, fully and legally approved by the FDA for use during pregnancy to prevent miscarriages, manufactured by drug companies, prescribed by doctors.

There is a strange footnote to the Dieckmann study. In 1978 two American researchers took another look at Dieckmann's figures and concluded that he had missed something: not only did DES not prevent miscarriages, as his study had shown, but, they claimed, a proper analysis of his numbers showed that DES *caused* miscarriages.

Yvonne Brackbill, Ph.D., who holds joint appointments in the departments of psychology and obstetrics-gynecology at the University of Florida, in Gainesville, and Heinz W. Berendes, M.D., a leading researcher in the National Institute of Child Health and Human Development, a part of the National Institutes of Health, concluded that women in Dieckmann's study who had taken DES had nearly twice as many spontaneous abortions as women in the study who had been given the placebo. Additionally, they found that women who had been given DES in the study had four times as many neonatal deaths (deaths of infants in the first four weeks after birth) as did the women who had taken the placebo.

Their findings for this drug, so widely used in America, were significant—but they couldn't get their paper published here. It was published in England, in the September 2, 1978, issue of *Lancet*, a medical publication aimed at Great Britain's doctors.

Why wasn't their paper published here? The *New England Journal of Medicine* reviewer stated:

> The observations appear to be correct, but it is not clear what is to be learned from them. Evidently the practice of [DES use in pregnancy] has ended, largely because of the carcinogenic effect and secondarily because of its ineffectiveness . . . Is there a lesson to be learned from the unfortunate experience? . . . Were there other reasons for failure of the Dieckmann paper to end the practice? . . . Did it fail because of personalities? Were the Dieckmann colleagues unable to compete with the prominence of the famous Smiths? . . . Were reputations or commercial interests at stake? If the authors have some special insight into the episode, the present report might be expanded into a much more informative one.

The second rejection of the paper came from the *American Journal of Obstetrics and Gynecology*, the journal that had published the Smiths's work and Dieckmann's rebuttal to it. The reviewer challenged the findings and conclusions of the reevaluation, although a leading federal government statistician had confirmed them.

The upshot was that the final medical coda to the battle of DES effectiveness and safety was never heard in this country. It was heard in England, where DES was only rarely used during pregnancy.

6

GOVERNMENT APPROVAL AND THE MARKETING OF DES

Just after the turn of the century Upton Sinclair, a young social reformer with anger in his heart and a way with words, took a look at the stockyards in Chicago—the greed of the packing companies, the unsanitary conditions under which table meat was prepared—and wrote a trailblazing novel about what he saw, *The Jungle*. Although he couched his findings in fictional terms, in part for greater impact, in part for legal protection, the power of his observations was such that only months after the book's 1906 publication, Congress passed the Food and Drug Act.

The standards of the Act, requiring certain showing of purity, strength, and consistency, remained fundamentally unchanged for the next three decades, although some critics inside and outside the government said that science and industry were changing faster than regulators could handle the changes. That criticism stayed in the realm of the esoteric until 1937, when approximately one hundred Americans, many of them children, died after taking a legally licensed drug called Sulfanilamide. That drug had met existing standards for purity and strength but had not been tested for safety, since that was not required. The next year, in 1938, a major change was made in FDA regulations: drugs now had to be shown to be safe before they could be licensed for use. Nineteen thirty-eight was also the year Dodds synthesized DES. Sociologist Susan E. Bell writes in her Brandeis thesis that DES was the first drug that was not life-saving to be tested under the new standard.

That testing was something that sections of the drug industry probably did not mind. The drug industry had been growing and changing along with the country. It had long since ceased being a supplier of medications "guaranteed" to cure baldness, lumbago, the common cold, and dyspepsia. The newly emerging ethical drug companies, the ones making prescription drugs that could be used only by a doctor's order, probably wanted the U.S. government seal of approval on their products. These companies, including all the ones that later made DES, made their money by convincing doctors to prescribe their products and persuading pharmacists to stock the drugs. Government approval gave ethical backing to the products, and that helped sales.

There was also a new development in American industry, which came along like a giant wave that would eventually carry the boat called DES along. Prior to the 1930s there were many "Mom and Pop" drug companies around the country, making products that had a local following or were marketed by some of the bigger firms, usually located "back east."

But the introduction of sulfa drugs in 1935 changed all that. For almost the first time physicians had a wide variety of products to use against a wide variety of common bacterial diseases. These drugs were not "Mom and Pop" varieties but ethical drug products marketed by the major manufacturers, who were fiercely competing to consolidate their markets. The short time between the administration of such a drug and the "cure" of the underlying problem prompted the use of the term "miracle drug." That phrase had been in somewhat more limited use for the previous decade, ever since the discovery in 1921 of insulin. When researchers such as Karnaky reported seeing cramping and bleeding stop in just seconds after DES was administered, it too began to be regarded as a miracle drug.

With the establishment by the federal government of its first drug industry regulatory agency, and with new and potentially profitable drugs coming along all the time, the drug companies banded together to form a lobbying voice to ensure that their side of various issues was heard. One year after the FDA was established in 1906, the American Association of Pharmaceutical Chemists, a lobbying group, set up offices in Washington in order to represent the industry point of view to regulators. Another such lobby group was the National Association of Manufacturers of Medicinal Products, founded in 1912 and renamed the American Drug Manufacturers in 1916. These two friendly factions— the pharmaceutical people and the drug manufacturers—combined forces in 1958 to form the powerful Pharmaceutical Manufacturers Association.

It should be pointed out, however, that there were no lobbying groups representing the consumer. Until Ralph Nader gave a voice and a presence to the consumers, they had no real voice.

Looking back, it can be seen that DES caused great excitement in the medical and scientific communities almost from the moment of its existence. Cheap, effective by mouth, duplicating all the powers of natural estrogens—that's what it looked like to scientists. But the drug companies could not have failed to note something else: it existed, unpatented, in the public domain. That meant its formula was available for anyone who wanted it, without charge. The companies incurred few research costs and paid no licensing fees or royalties. Aside from production and marketing costs, most traditional overhead costs were eliminated, thus offering the potential for high profit margins.

Dozens of companies were immediately interested in DES. The need was there for a good medical product with its potency; the market was there. Squibb executives wined and dined Karl John Karnaky in order to get him to use DES. Squibb sent DES to George and Olive Smith on request. Squibb supplied DES for the 1940 animal studies by Northwestern University researchers Greene, Burrill, and Ivy showing that animals exposed *in utero* had anatomical and structural abnormalities. Squibb supplied DES to Alfred University scientists Burdick and Vedder for studies showing that DES caused the ova of test animals to "disintegrate," thereby preventing pregnancies. The New Jersey-based company also sent free samples to practicing doctors in New York, Los Angeles, Boston, Detroit, and other cities.

Despite my repeated requests, Squibb officials were never available for comment.

In Indianapolis, Eli Lilly launched its own research program and assigned employee Don Carlos Hines to watch new developments in the field and keep in touch with all the top people in the field. Lilly sent DES samples to top people in Birmingham, Louisville, Kansas City, Sykesville (Maryland), and other cities.

Within months of learning of its existence here, in fact, American drug companies were pounding on federal doors, seeking an OK to market it for traditional estrogen-related matters, mainly those involving menopause. But at the same time, conservative medical people were publicly warning that this potent new drug might be too risky to put on the market, because its long-range effects were unknown. The December 23, 1939, issue of the *Journal of the American Medical Association* (JAMA) contained an editorial entitled, "Estrogen Therapy—A Warning." "Regarding conflicting reports about DES," the editorial stated, "apparently a thorough investigation of this compound is in order before it can be prescribed for routine therapy . . . the possibility of carcinoma induced by estrogens cannot be ignored . . . it appears likely the medical profession may be importuned to prescribe to patients large doses of high potency estrogens, such as stilbestrol, because of the ease of administration of these preparations."

In the same issue of JAMA the Council on Pharmacy and Chemistry, an advisory group of practicing physicians and scholars, published three separate reports on DES, all of which mentioned worrisome side effects, such as nausea. Regarding menopausal use, one report stated: "A variety of toxic effects were observed. A number of these, such as nausea, vomiting, abdominal distress, anorexia, and diarrhea, were associated with the gastrointestinal tract, and have been reported by other workers. They were frequent enough to alarm not only the patients but also the investigators." The authors of that report included Ephraim Shorr, M.D. (who, as an FDA adviser, several years later recommended against federal approval of DES) and George N. Papanicolaou, M.D., who had developed the widely used Pap smear technique for judging the health of the vagina.

The Council itself concluded: "Because the product is so potent and because the possibility of harm must be recognized, the Council is of the opinion that it should not be recognized for general use or for inclusion in New and Nonofficial Remedies [a category for experimental drugs] at the present time and that its use by the general medical profession should not be undertaken until further studies have led to a better understanding of the proper functions of the drug."

Only four months later, in the April 20, 1940, issue, the editors of JAMA issued another editorial on the subject of estrogens, which included DES. Having noted that some doctors were using smaller doses of estrogens to treat some patients and so avoid toxic side effects, the editorial stated: "It would be unwise to consider that there is safety in using small doses of estrogens, since it is quite possible that the same harm may be obtained through the use of small doses of estrogen if they are maintained over a long period."

Whether those concerns were recognized by the medical profession and the drug industry depends on your point of view. Consumers who have been harmed, or fear they may be harmed in the future, say the warnings were not heeded. The drug companies say that the effects that later turned out to be associated with DES could not have been anticipated at the time. Despite whatever additional tests they say they made, they always kept marketing the drug.

One thing is clear, and that is that the drug companies were pushing mightily to get DES approved for use. Squibb and Lilly were not the only companies sending samples of DES to doctors around the country. Such firms as Abbott Laboratories, Sharp & Dohme, and the Upjohn Company were doing it too, according to documents filed in various lawsuits.

This early use was considered a means of "testing," for which formal approval was not then needed. The "testing" would be used as proof that the drug should be made widely available, through drug stores, for prescription use. This was a traditional method of testing drugs: sending free samples to practitioners, advising them how the drug should be used, asking them to distribute the drug to patients, then requesting information about its effects. In theory this is the kind of situation that benefits everyone: the drug companies get information, the patient gets a free sample, and the doctor is passing on the latest medical advance to his patients, who look to him for guidance and help. It is also, incidentally, a good example of the close working relationship between drug companies and practicing physicians.

So the push was on to get DES approved for widespread use. In 1940 about a dozen U.S. drug companies filed applications with the FDA to market DES. They were Abbott Laboratories, Ayerst, McKenna & Company, George A. Breon & Company, Charles E. Frosst & Company, Eli Lilly, Merck, William S. Merrell Company, Sharp & Dohme, Inc., E. R. Squibb & Sons, Upjohn, Winthrop Chemical, and Wyeth Laboratories.

But FDA officials, concerned about all the controversy in the field—which in part had been brought to their attention by the JAMA editorials—let the word out that the applications were going to be turned down, according to federal documents filed in court. The companies had two choices: they could protest and request that hearings be held, or they could quietly withdraw their applications, regroup, and come back to fight another day.

If hearings were held, the press might attend. Since the only standard of the day involved safety, public discussions about the carcinogenic qualities of DES and of all estrogens could provide the kind of publicity nobody needed. Withdrawing the applications might work out best: it would be quiet, everything would be discreet, and until the drug companies could figure out how to get their way, they could avoid confusion about the qualities of DES.

The applications were withdrawn by the drug companies by telegram on December 30, 1940, and formally approved for withdrawal by the FDA on January 17, 1941.

That is the way Washington worked then, and that is the way Washington works now. Quietly, subtly, with nods and understandings, assurances and unwritten agreements, it sets up a revolving door that moves people out of government and into the industries they once regulated, out of regulated industries and into the seats of power.

Carson P. Frailey, executive vice-president of the American Drug Manufacturers Association, had been an industry official since the 1920s. It is *not* important that he was present during the presidencies of Calvin Coolidge, Herbert Hoover, and Franklin Delano Roosevelt; it *is* important that he was present during all the years *bureaucrats and civil servants* under those presidents were in power. Career administrators are the ones who make the evaluations for their bosses; the bosses are usually political appointees, and as such may well be gone after the next presidential elections. Lobbyists make it part of their job to know all the people in the middle levels of government, the ones who will be around regardless of which party is in power. This is also true for large corporations and consumer groups.

After the drug companies withdrew their applications, and at the suggestion of an FDA official who wanted to simplify the process of receiving data on a commonly made product from a large number of companies, the firms decided to pool their resources for the creation of a master file on DES designed to win the government seal of approval in the next round. They formed a committee of four member firms that would do the bulk of the work on behalf of all of them. The four companies whose members were on this committee were Lilly, Squibb, Winthrop Chemical Company, and Upjohn. Don Carlos Hines, a physician from Lilly, became head of the group, which, because of its size, became known as the Small Committee.

DES suited Eli Lilly & Company very well. Founded in 1874 by Colonel Eli Lilly, a civil war hero, Lilly was and is one of the largest pharmaceutical companies in the world. One of its specialties was making pills. It made at least half, and possibly 75 percent of all DES sold in this country, which it marketed under its own name and also sold in bulk to other firms—although, as nearly as anyone can tell, the true figures are cloaked behind more lawyers and lawsuits than have ever been involved in any other product-liability area in history. In one current lawsuit, Washington, D.C., attorney Aaron M. Levine cites Lilly figures showing the company made 716 million units of DES for all purposes from 1942 to 1971. Lilly attorneys state that the company does not know how many of its DES pills were used for the prevention of miscarriage and how many were used for other purposes.

The company's total sales in 1980 were $2.6 billion, nearly double the $1.23 billion net sales figure it rang up only five years earlier. For most of the preceding decade, and apparently for most years prior to that, its annual rate of increased sales was at least 10 percent—the type of figure that delights financial analysts and is attributed to the company's tough, aggressive, and effective marketing.

In a special promotional booklet put out to commemorate its hundred-year anniversary, the company stated that in 1975 it had spent the impressive sum of $104 million on research and development of new drugs, chemicals, and products—but more than twice that, $208 million, on marketing those products.

And marketing is what Eli Lilly & Company is very good at, possibly as good as any other firm in its field. Its army of salesmen—in the 1940s and 1950s it numbered as many as 400—would fan out across the country, calling on physicians and retail pharmacists. According to its little known in-house publications, Lilly sales representatives in 1949—eight years after DES had been approved for nonpregnancy uses and two years after its OK for pregnancy—made 800,000 calls on America's doctors and one million calls on its retail pharamacists.

To doctors the company (like other drug companies) offered free samples, medical booklets, and an assortment of gizmos and gadgets for the doctor's personal and professional uses, all of them imprinted with its own logo. To pharmacists Lilly offered incentive plans for buying Lilly products and selling Lilly brands—price breaks on gross purchases, discounts on loss leaders.

Lilly has always set out to be the complete drug house, the firm that makes every product a physician would need. Lilly prides itself on making "everything for the physician's medical bag," Robert H. Furman, M.D., the company's current medical director, said in an interview. Depending upon what medical school a doctor graduated from, Lilly might have given him the medical bag too, as several doctors—who still have their Lilly-donated black bags—can confirm.

The giant company did more than simply make chemicals—they packaged them for easy consumer use. In Lilly's case, a major interest was pills. In 1890 Lilly engineers designed the world's first semiautomatic capsule-making machines, giving the firm an edge over its competition. In 1932 the company purchased the world's first fully automatic capsule-making machines. By 1948, the year after DES was approved for use during pregnancy, the company was making eleven million capsules each day for all types of medicine.

DES was synthesized in 1938, and only months later it was known in England that the drug could be taken orally in capsule form, a form of preparation in which Lilly specialized.

In order to get DES on the market, the job of the Small Committee (headed by a Lilly employee) was to convince FDA regulators that DES was safe for specified uses—the only standard in effect at the time.

It was at this time that J. A. Morrell of Squibb collected 257 articles on DES showing the drug's use in clinical situations. The emphasis on "clinical" is important, because clinical uses are the uses to which a doctor in his office would put the drug, rather than uses restricted to laboratory test animals. Stressing the clinical impact of DES also kept attention away from the theoretical concerns and published animal studies showing that as an estrogen, DES was a member of a well known cancer-causing family.

The lobbying groups also urged physicians, according to court papers, to write to the FDA regarding their own clinical experience with DES. According to one court file, the FDA had only two full-time staff physicians equipped to deal with reports on more than five thousand patients who had been given DES.

As these massive and largely positive reports were arriving at FDA headquarters on C Street, the members of the Small Committee continued meeting. On January 28, 1941, eleven days after the FDA had officially permitted the companies to withdraw their applications, drug industry lobbyist Carson P. Frailey hosted a 10 A.M. meeting of committee members at the Washington Hotel.

Five months later the industry's lobbying wizardry and the reports from physicians across the country had apparently had their effect. On May 12, 1941, Frailey sent similar letters to the Small Committee members: "The time now seems propitious to suggest that you re-file

[your] new drug application for stilbestrol. I am making no commitments that the application will be permitted to become effective, but the suggestion offered has official background."

During this time the FDA considered reports from 54 doctors, using DES supplied by the drug companies, and only 4 of the physicians felt DES should not be approved.

On September 19, 1941, DES was officially approved by the FDA for use in four types of treatment: gonorrheal vaginitis (a vaginal infection that can lead to serious complications), menopausal symptoms (including so-called "hot flashes" caused by a natural decrease of estrogens), senile vaginitis (in postmenopausal women this inflammation can lead to an ulceration of the vaginal cells), and to prevent lactation in women who had recently given birth. It was not approved for any purposes that the FDA felt had not been proven safe, including amenorrhea and dysmenorrhea.

Once it was approved for the four limited purposes, the law permitted it to be used by physicians for other purposes, in an experimental capacity. According to FDA officials, the agency does not interfere with a doctor's right to practice medicine, even though, as in the case of DES, he might be using a legal drug for a purpose for which it had not been approved.

It is at this point, in 1941, immediately after the FDA's initial approval of DES for use with menopausal women, that the interest in using DES to prevent miscarriages accelerated. It was used first by Karl John Karnaky in Houston, with results published in 1942, then with Priscilla White and the Smiths's diabetic patients in Boston, then in the early trials conducted by George and Olive Smith, published in 1946.

DES was approved for use in preventing miscarriages in 1947, although it had been widely used on what was called an experimental basis before that. There was far less intense lobbying in order to get this additional approval, as far as can be gleaned from the public record. DES was already approved for some purposes, and with this new drug application, it could be approved for another. The federal government, in its capacity as a watchdog agency, had no different standards from the medical profession as a whole. Although DES would be given to pregnant women, there were no tests on the long-range impact the drug might have on the children. One report had been conducted on children born to women in the Smiths's study, but it examined children only at the age of six months, and had found no noticeable differences between them and non-DES-exposed children.

The Greene, Burrill, and Ivy studies—showing harm to the reproductive systems of test animals exposed *in utero*—might have provided an alert to study the reproductive capacity of the first generation of DES children, but the focus of the time was on the mothers, not on the children. No one ever demanded that the studies be done; no one ever did those studies. Other studies showing the carcinogenic powers of DES might also have been taken as warnings, but were not. "It was interesting information about the actions of the drug," Lilly counsel Raymond Rauch said in an interview.

The Lilly attitude toward its relationship with the government can be gleaned from an in-house brochure the corporation published for its employees around the world. There is no reason to think that this drug company's attitude on the subject of government relations was different from that of other corporations in other fields. Although published in the March 1953 issue of the *Lilly Review*, it embodies ideas that existed a decade earlier and still exist today throughout the corridors of American enterprise.

The article states:

> [The FDA] has managed to gain the respect of private business—no small accomplishment for a government agency . . . Briefly, the FDA's job is to protect the general public from unsafe drugs, contaminated food, and harmful cosmetics. To most Lilly people—deeply conscious of our own efforts to insure quality and accuracy—such protection might seem unnecessary. But to the eleven hundred FDA workers who confiscate twenty-seven tons of putrid food a day and have ordered many a dangerous drug off the market, nothing is safe until exhaustive tests prove it so . . . The FDA, with its galaxy of rules and policies, has—on occasion—vexed many a hard-driving businessman. When pinned down to basic facts, however, most Lilly people who know the FDA agree that it does a necessary job in an effective manner. One Lilly man who has dealt with the agency nearly every day . . . summed it up this way: "We don't always agree with the FDA, but I don't recall the time that our differences weren't settled reasonably. They act in the interest of the entire pharmaceutical industry, and what's good for the industry is usually good for us."

A picture in the same article showed a Lilly employee ensuring quality-control standards for a batch of antibiotics. The caption read: "Every lot of most antibiotics from every manufacturer is tested in Washington. One in two hundred is rejected for sterility or potency reasons. FDA regulations are subject to open hearings, often follow industry recommendations."

Why the great interest in expanding the use of DES to prevent miscarriages? Because there was nothing else as cheap, as easy to take, or seemingly, as effective. And there was the market: by 1947 the war was over, the suburbs were expanding, and the baby boom was in full swing. In 1941, when DES received its first limited approval, babies were being born at the rate of 20.3 for every 1,000 people. By 1947, when DES was approved for use in pregnancy, babies were being born at the rate of 26.6 per 1,000 people, a 31-percent increase. And the 1947 baby birth rate was the highest this country had seen since 1920. Moreover, if one out of every five pregnancies ended in a miscarriage, then four mothers delivered for every one who did not. And if having babies was part of the national mood, then saving pregnancies was a part of the national purpose.

The Eli Lilly company implicitly emphasized this to its sales force in a 1948 in-house publication: "Last year . . . a live baby was born in a hospital *every 15 seconds* [their italics] (more than two million). It's a great market ready and waiting for a salesman who can sell—service and satisfaction. Tried it lately?"

E. R. Squibb & Sons may have sent its executives around the country in the early days, getting researchers to test DES, but by the time DES had been approved in 1947 for pregnancy use, as well as menopausal uses, the Lilly marketing juggernaut, as far as can be told from federal documents and court papers, ran rings around them and every other company competing directly with them.

With its army of as many as four hundred salesmen nationwide making daily or at least weekly calls on doctors and pharmacists, Lilly was able to keep its products active and used. One year before DES was approved for use in pregnancy, the April 1946 issue of the *Lilly Review* ran a photograph of a gloved hand holding an enormous scooper full of white DES powder used for making 25-milligram tablets of DES, which could be used for relief of menopausal problems or, as was done later, during pregnancy. The May 1948 issue of the *Lilly Wholesalesman*, an informational brochure for Lilly representatives, urged salesmen: "DEAL YOURSELF IN . . . play a winning hand—the LILLY DETAIL PROGRAM for May. Here it is. *To Druggists:* . . . Diethylstilbestrol. *To You:* Turn on the steam—and discover how good business really is."

Lilly could charge $7.51 for a bottle of 25-milligram pills, knowing a druggist was more likely to fill a prescription with it because he could make a higher profit with Lilly products than with other brands of DES, which sold for as little as $1.10 for the same bottle.

When Lilly detail men got inside a doctor's office, they could leave him preprinted forms on which he could order DES. One part of the form was labeled "For Office Record . . . Dosage Schedule for Diethyl-stilbestrol in Accidents of Pregnancy" and contained a preprinted dosage schedule that followed the Smiths's recommendations. Another form was printed for the patient's use, showing how much DES was to be taken. At the bottom of that form was the helpful reminder: "Date of next office visit." The third part of the form was a prescription blank to be filled out by the doctor, handed to the patient, and given to the druggist to be filled with DES in either 5-milligram or 25-milligram "Enseals" capsules, made only by Lilly. This blank, with an enormous "Rx" printed at the top, also contained a line at the bottom for the doctor's signature, next to the letters "M.D."

In case a doctor wanted to read some printed literature about DES, the company printed, and detail men gave away, small brochures. One of them was called "Diethylstilbestrol in Accidents of Pregnancy." In itself, this shows the wide use of which DES was being put. Many of the early studies favorable to DES had concentrated on accidents of late pregnancy in women with a history of miscarriages. This brochure, however, included everyone. "Recent work has indicated that diethyl-stilbestrol may have value as an aid in prevention of certain types of accidents of pregnancy, such as threatened abortion, habitual abortion," and for use with diabetic women, it stated. The brochure cited work by the Smiths, Karnaky, and others, as well as "Rosenblum and Melinkoff [who] have published their observations [of] an unselected group of ninety-six patients with threatened or habitual abortion."

Rosenblum and Melinkoff were the Los Angeles physicians who had also raised the four thoughtful questions about the then unknown implications of DES use, including the question about whether DES might be carcinogenic when used in such large doses. The Lilly brochure did not include those questions.

In 1951 Lilly published *De Re Medica* (Concerning Things of Medicine), which was edited by Don Carlos Hines, M.D., the Lilly official who had served as head of the Small Committee. The textbook-type publication discussed a wide variety of medical matters. On the subject of miscarriages the publication stated: "Recent evidence indicates that the percentage of cases salvaged can be considerably increased by the oral administration of diethylstilbestrol. Dosage is not entirely settled, but an effective schedule seems to be 25 mg. as soon as the diagnosis is made, followed by 5 mg. every fifteen minutes or 25 mg. every hour until bleeding or cramps or both have ceased. After this, 5 mg. are given three times daily. It is difficult to determine when the drug can be safely discontinued. There is no harm in continuing it through the thirty-sixth week."

An accompanying table showing the DES program recommended by the Smiths was entitled "Dosage Schedule for Oral Administration of Diethylstilbestrol in Prevention of Accidents of Pregnancy." In other words, DES was here being recommended to prevent miscarriages from occurring, not simply treating them when they threatened.

The section on cancer identified estrogens as being capable of producing cancer under certain conditions. DES, of course, was a synthetic estrogen.

During the 1950s the controlled studies by Dieckmann, Ferguson, Crowder, and others were published, showing in each of those reports that women given DES did not have fewer miscarriages than those who hadn't been given the drug. A Lilly brochure published in 1961, covering all uses of DES, however, did not mention those studies. The brochure did quote a few negative DES studies, including the one by Robinson and Shettles stating that all those authors "do not feel that hormonal therapy is of significant benefit in the . . . treatment of threatened or repeated abortion."

Actually, the Robinson and Shettles paper had concluded: "The present study indicates that diethylstilbestrol is, in fact, a dismal failure in the treatment of threatened abortion."

When William J. Dieckmann, M.D., at the University of Chicago, had begun his controlled, double-blind study of DES, he had used DES tablets purchased from the Eli Lilly company. He bought $69,000 worth of DES and identical placebo pills from Lilly for the reduced price of $23,300. Dieckmann obtained a $34,836 federal grant to pay for the pills and for technical assistance.

But in its literature Lilly left out his conclusions.

Lilly officials today attack Dieckmann's methods and what they claim was the way in which some patients were eliminated from the study before they had delivered. "We were not recommending this product for normal pregnant women, and that's what he studied," Raymond Rauch said. Asked why no studies were ever done to refute

Dieckmann's findings, using methods that were closer to what the company claims it was recommending, Lilly executive Robert H. Furman, M.D., replied, "No studies were done to refute Dieckmann because his study was flawed."

And as long as the drug couldn't hurt, traditional business practice—and medical practice—was to keep using it. One would think that the thalidomide disaster of the 1960s should have resulted in further testing of DES. In 1962 the U.S. Congress had changed the Food, Drug, and Cosmetic Act of 1938. Until 1962, drugs only had to be shown to be safe to get FDA approval. After 1962, new drugs had to be shown to be effective as well as safe before they could get FDA approval. Drugs on the market in 1962 could be "grandfathered" in, but they would have to be retested. The federal retesting of DES indicated that it was "possibly effective" but that substantial additional retesting would be needed to prove it.

Lilly officials in 1968 removed pregnancy use from the list of "Indications" it published in its package inserts, and it inserted a warning: "Because of possible adverse reactions on the fetus, the risk of estrogen therapy should be weighed against the possible benefits when diethylstilbestrol is considered for use in a known pregnancy." This commendable warning, however, does not explicitly tell the doctor not to use DES, only to consider the consequences. Nor were restrictions for pregnancy use listed in the "Contraindications" section of the package insert, as they could have been. Nor did Lilly stop selling the drug for other purposes, or instruct (as far as is known) its sales force not to sell it for the use in pregnancy that had been advocated for at least fifteen years; nor did it stop selling DES in bulk to other companies.

Legally it did not have to do any of these things, because there were as yet no known negative effects on women who took it or the children born to them. And although medical standards and laws had changed in the years since DES first came on the scene, Lilly and the other drug companies were under no obligation to retest it or limit its sales.

In late 1971, after a medical report was published linking DES and vaginal cancer in daughters exposed *in utero*, the FDA withdrew its approval for DES use during pregnancy, and so pregnancy use was listed under the "Contraindications" section of descriptive drug information.

In 1972 Eli Lilly & Company began giving research grants to university and other investigators across the country interested in finding out how the drug worked, as well as screening some of the exposed people. According to court papers filed in Washington, D.C., from 1972 to

1981, Lilly spent $1,240,552 for research by outside investigators. That type of research could have been done before the drug was marketed, but society didn't demand it, and the company didn't have to do it.

As will be shown in another chapter, an unprecedented number of lawsuits against drug companies have developed in recent years regarding DES use. Lilly has always vigorously defended its own conduct. Company officials today justify the use of DES during pregnancy as having been consistent with the most up-to-date medical information available in the 1940s and 1950s. During a three-hour interview, two top executives made these additional comments:

"No one could have predicted" the various problems that have been associated with DES use, Lilly medical director Robert H. Furman, M.D., said. DES was originally looked at "reasonably carefully ... Out of Harvard comes substantial creditable evidence for people at risk of losing a pregnancy ... I'm not aware of any clear-cut refutation of [Olive Smith's] data ... If this occurred today consumer organizations would be hailing this as a ... great breakthrough in keeping medical costs down ... In all probability [DES] would pass [federal requirements for safety and efficacy]. With the proper selection of the proper patient population, I feel reasonably confident that efficacy could be clearly established. That's a professional opinion, it's not a scientific fact."

Raymond Rauch said: "The marketing people didn't have the market for accidents of pregnancy on their minds [in the late 1940s], they were thinking of antibiotics, that's where the money was. Our total sales for all DES used for all purposes was two and a half million to three million dollars, from 1947 to 1971"—a small sum for a billion-dollar company. "The doctors I talked to didn't think those animal studies had any applicability to humans at the time, and I'm not sure they have today. In 1970 nobody saw any need to do additional studies in animals, because they weren't seeing anything wrong in people ... If we did the tests today, without knowing [about the 1971 cancer report from Massachusetts General Hospital], the answer would very likely be yes"—that Lilly would market DES for pregnancy use, he said. "You can never tell in any given case whether a drug had anything to do with a condition ... pregnancy probably is the most complicated of human events."

Regarding drug use in pregnancy, Robert H. Furman, M.D., stated, "You have to take a risk-versus-benefit analysis."

The smaller drug companies often did not have sales forces that could call on physicians. They had to resort to advertising in medical journals. One DES ad appeared in the *American Journal of Obstetrics and Gynecology* in the mid-1950s. It showed a picture of a plump baby, finger to mouth, looking over his shoulder and saying, "Really?" The advertising copy answered his question: "Yes, desPLEX to prevent abortion, miscarriage and premature labor . . . recommended for routine prophylaxis [prevention] in ALL pregnancies." The ad was published by the Grant Chemical Company of Brooklyn, which made desPLEX tablets containing DES and vitamins B and C. A scholarly reference in the ad was to a January 1954 article in the *American Journal of Surgery*, by Eduardo F. Peña, M.D., of Miami. The second paragraph of Peña's article states; "For this purpose [to prevent miscarriages and avoid pregnancy problems caused by a lack of vitamins] a convenient combination of estrogen and vitamins is found in desPLEX tablets." The pills had been supplied by Grant Chemical Company.

The financial benefit to marketing DES in the midst of the baby boom was such that E. R. Squibb & Sons was able to ignore a letter from one of its own detail men quoting New York City physicians who said the drug didn't work. The letter, dated November 22, 1950, said that two New York physicians disputed the conclusions of George and Olive Smith and that Stilbetin, Squibb's version of DES, caused "more missed abortions [miscarriages] than any other form of therapy." Squibb officials have declined comment.

Physicians did not need to rely on drug company detail men to inform them of DES. Several I talked to said their patients came in and asked for it by name, or for something they had read about in popular magazines which they could not identify by name but which could only be DES.

DES was not a subject confined to the pages of the medical magazines. The popular press also mentioned it, usually in articles on miscarriage.

In the December 1949 *Good Housekeeping*, Maxine Davis wrote in her article "Miscarriage": "Every woman who has a miscarriage is shocked and disappointed. Many are frightened. This experience is, of course, unfortunate; but it is far from infrequent and should not be too alarming." She added cautiously, "Sometimes doctors use stilbestrol, which stimulates estrogenic activity, to prevent threatened miscarriage . . . Sometimes physicians prescribe progesterone, or a combination of progesterone and estrogen. The use of these hormones or stilbestrol is new and highly controversial. Conservative obstetricians feel that their value is as yet far from proven."

In the November 1950 *Woman's Home Companion*, J. D. Ratcliff wrote in his article called "Miscarriage": "Today, fortunately, physicians are far better qualified to handle and prevent miscarriages than they were even a few years ago. But are you aware of the progress they have made? . . . Fortunately, physicians are now armed with tests to detect a shortage of essential progesterone. By injection or by mouth they can supply additional hormones—often with dramatic success . . . The miracle drugs that have tumbled from the laboratories in such heartening profusion recently have markedly reduced the number of miscarriages. . . ."

There was an anti-DES article in the May 1954 issue of *McCall's*. Jane Whitbread and Vivian Cadden wrote of a woman who had taken DES as a last resort in 1949 and carried that pregnancy only four months. Then she was treated by a physician who put her on a regimen of vitamins, including vitamin C, and specifically kept her away from DES and other hormones. She had a baby. (Recent research, however, has indicated that vitamin C may be harmful to the developing fetus.)

Other articles and columns talked favorably about hormones in general, or stilbestrol in particular, as being a part of the new era of medical care. Those popular pieces reflected much contemporary belief about pregnancy aids, and, in keeping with the optimistic spirit of the times, failed to even raise the question of potential risks.

In the August 1959 issue of *Reader's Digest* was an article written by Edith L. Potter, M.D., a staff pathologist at the University of Chicago. Her article began: "Each day some 2500 American women pregnant for less than six months lose their babies through miscarriage." She wrote that "there are many causes of miscarriage" and that "the method of treatment of a woman who has had several miscarriages may vary widely."

Then she stated, "Some obstetricians report excellent results with progesterone or other hormones." While that implies that some obstetricians don't report excellent results, it doesn't state it, and her article contained no reference to the article published six years earlier showing that DES, a synthetic hormone, as used by William J. Dieckmann and his colleagues, did not prevent miscarriages.

Regardless of the marketing genius of Eli Lilly & Company, or any of the other nearly three hundred firms that made or distributed DES for nearly thirty years, it would have been a complete commercial flop if it hadn't been for two other factors in the DES phenomenon. Drug companies may make a drug, but unless doctors are willing to prescribe it and patients are willing to take it, it will fail.

Drug companies wanted to supply a product that might help people and also make money. Their actions followed the advice of some researchers (though not all). But what about the doctors who dealt on a day-to-day basis with pregnant women, doctors who had the opportunity to read the debate going on in the medical journals, the claims for its effectiveness, the claims for its uselessness, the concerns or assurances about its cancer-causing potential? It has not been easy finding physicians willing to talk at all, much less talk on the record. Several, including several strong anti-DES people, simply refused to talk for attribution and would not give their reasons. But I did meet two thoughtful physicians who helped put DES into its social and medical context.

William G. Karow, M.D., is with the Southern California Fertility Institute in Los Angeles. His medical specialty is infertility, and he used DES widely in his practice. On his own initiative he notified thousands of former patients and their daughters about their DES exposure when the first reports came out. He is also the coauthor, with psychologist June Machover Reinisch, of a paper on the psychological influence that DES has after it is administered *in utero*.

"The heartaches of infertility include, on the average, sixty-six months of marriage, thirty-six months of trying to conceive, and then a pregnancy that is lost. Therefore people involved with infertility were willing to try anything," he said.

Karow was a young medical school student in the 1950s when DES was being most strongly advocated by its medical champions. "I remember a professor once, who every six months or so would talk about its effectiveness. He would say he had a drug that was so good he just couldn't keep it away from his patients."

As a young physician (he received his M.D. in 1955), Karow respected the stature of DES advocates. "We were very impressed by Karnaky. He would go to medical conferences and pass out article after article on DES. He had charts he put up, showing its effectiveness. I remember one article that said eleven women had lost a total of forty-four children until DES came along, and then they had eight babies between them. And there was a sound physiological concept as to why it should work. That concept was advocated by the Smiths, the leading endocrinologists in the field of obstetrics-gynecology."

Across the country, in Alexandria, Virginia—just across the Potomac River from Washington—gynecologist George Speck, M.D., also used DES with some patients who were having difficulty in getting pregnant.

"Look at it this way: a woman comes in, she's trying to get pregnant after a lot of trying. She gets pregnant, she misses her period, and she's

scared to death [that she'll have a miscarriage]. What do you do? If you
follow the University of Chicago school, you tell her to go to bed. If the
pregnancy's a good one, fine; if it's bad, it'll abort. Okay, she loses the
pregnancy, with all the anguish that involves. She gets pregnant again,
and starts staining. Do you put her on her back or say, 'Here's a drug
we've been using. If the pregnancy's defective, you'll lose it. But if it's
good, this may help you.' She goes back thinking, Here's a man who
wants to help. Psychologically she has a lift, and therapeutically she
may be helped. Even if you gave her a sugar pill, that might help, but
you can't be callous. She's searching for something, and we felt possibly
this might help."

Among Washington-area doctors George Speck has an outstanding
reputation for helping women have babies, and I was referred to him by
one of his patients, Mary Patton, who had taken DES after some fertility difficulties and whose daughter Nola is now sixteen and has not experienced any problems.

"There were too many variables in the Dieckmann study" for him to
stop prescribing DES because of it, Speck said. "It didn't really show us
anything. But we always come back to the same thing: You're a doctor
in private practice, you become involved with your patients. You want
to help your patient, and you find a drug that [seems] to offer help."

7

DISCOVERY OF A RARE FORM OF VAGINAL CANCER IN SOME DES DAUGHTERS

On the Fourth of July 1967 there were fireworks, tennis, softball games, swimming, and laughter when sixteen-year-old Shelley, who was at a New England summer camp, noticed some vaginal bleeding. She was sent almost immediately down to Massachusetts General Hospital in Boston, where Howard Ulfelder, M.D., diagnosed her as having an exceedingly rare form of vaginal cancer called clear-cell adenocarcinoma.

Shelley was the third young girl Ulfelder had seen in the previous three years with clear-cell adenocarcinoma, which had until then been seen only in women past the menopause, and never in girls so young. After seeing Shelley, Ulfelder remembers, "My nurse reports I came out of my office shaking my head and saying, 'There must be some explanation for this explosion.' "

On July 25, 1967, Ulfelder performed a radical hysterectomy and vaginectomy on Shelley, removing her uterus and vagina and replacing the vagina through a skin-graft procedure. Eighteen months later, in early 1969, Ulfelder, professor of gynecology at Harvard Medical School and deputy to the director for cancer affairs at Massachusetts General Hospital, was talking to Shelley's mother. Shelley was dressing in another room. They were in his first-floor office at Vincent Memorial Hospital, the location of Mass General's gynecologic service. As

Howard Ulfelder recalled it, "The mother said, 'I don't think I ever told you that when I was pregnant with Shelley the doctor put me on stilbestrol because I had lost one pregnancy. Could that have anything to do with it?'

"I said I didn't see how, but thanks anyway," Ulfelder recalled. "Then, when I asked the next mother, the mother of the second patient to come in, and she said yes, she had taken stilbestrol, I thought, My God . . ."

A colleague of Ulfelder's at the hospital, Arthur L. Herbst, M.D., later that year walked through the bitter cold of the Boston winter to knock on the door of another mother whose daughter also had had clear-cell adenocarcinoma. "You can stop your study," Herbst remembers the mother saying. "I took DES." Her daughter had died at the age of eighteen, in 1968. The cancer had appeared when she was fourteen years old.

Those initial linkages, a chance remark made to a skilled and scholarly physician, medical detective work by another, set off the chain of events that led to the original frightening association between DES and clear-cell adenocarcinoma in young girls whose mothers had taken the drug during pregnancy. That association was also the first in a chain of events that turned DES into one of the most influential medical phenomena of the times.

The years since have shown that vaginal cancer is a statistically small risk for exposed daughters, for whom there is a greater likelihood of having premature births or difficulties in getting pregnant than for other women. The ensuing years have also shown problems that DES sons should be aware of. But it was from that initial connection between DES taken by mothers and cancer in their daughters that the entire field of modern DES research began.

Howard Ulfelder saw his very first case of clear-cell adenocarcinoma in a young girl on May 11, 1966, when a patient was referred from her own doctor in Springfield, Massachusetts. The fifteen-year-old's physician had mentioned to Ulfelder at a medical conference earlier in the year that the girl had had the rare cancer. Ulfelder recalls he said he'd never heard of it appearing in a girl so young. It was his opinion that a watch-and-wait attitude ought to be taken regarding the teenager's fertility, which had not been terminated.

One year later another young woman with clear-cell adenocarcinoma was referred to the gynecology service. She was not as lucky: on May 18, 1967, she underwent a radical hysterectomy and vaginectomy, and doctors replaced her lost vagina with a surrogate one.

In July of 1967 Shelley came in.

Between 1966 and 1969 seven young women between fifteen and twenty-two years old with clear-cell adenocarcinoma of the vagina were seen by Ulfelder and two associates, Arthur L. Herbst, M.D., and David C. Poskanzer, M.D., who had joined him in trying to solve the puzzle. A twenty-year-old woman was treated for the same thing at another Boston hospital and was added to their study.

Howard Ulfelder is a thoughtful and quiet man who received his M.D. degree from Harvard in 1936. His inadvertent training for the DES crisis may have started in 1947, when, as an assistant to world-famous Harvard gynecologist Joe V. Meigs, M.D., he had seen a rare tumor called sarcoma botryoides in the vagina of a twenty-six-month-old baby. As in the cancer that turned out to be associated with DES, a thorough search of the existing medical literature found nothing of direct significance. New combinations of procedures were used, and the woman is today alive and well. But after that experience, Ulfelder was familiar with finding the unusual and dealing with it.

At a 1969 medical conference in San Francisco, Ulfelder heard of a similar case in California; and in October 1970 he read of yet another case in Mexico City. He wrote to the attending physicians of these additional cases and asked for details but purposely avoided mentioning DES. In both cases the physicians wrote back describing their patients and giving the information that each woman's mother had taken DES during pregnancy. These further cases placed the DES phenomenon on both a nationwide and international scale. "With those two extra cases I felt we had to come out with something so statistically significant that no one could argue" with them, said Ulfelder.

The Ulfelder group was insistent that any published reports linking DES to the group's recently published reports of clear-cell adenocarcinoma should be so solid that they could not be challenged. Ulfelder said he was concerned about what he described later as the "understandable unwillingness on the part of physicians, particularly those who had prescribed DES in the past" to accept the group's findings. Additionally, Ulfelder and others had no idea how widespread the phenomenon might be, because there were no estimates of the frequency of DES usage. They did not know to what degree, if at all, they were dealing with the start of an epidemic.

The Harvard team put together a clever and complex program with which to study the cancer phenomenon they had observed. It is worthwhile to look briefly at their methods, to see why a definitive association with cancer and DES could now be made. By contrast, the studies twenty years earlier claiming that DES was safe for pregnancy use look thin, even allowing for the improved statistical methods that had recently been developed.

To begin with, four controls—women who had been treated in as nearly identical a manner as possible, except that DES had not been used during their mothers' pregnancies—were chosen for each of the eight cancer cases. The controls were women born within five days of the eight cancer victims and in the same type of hospital setting (public or private). For example, if a cancer victim was born on the first day of a month and in a private hospital ward of a certain hospital, each of her four controls would have been born within five days of her birth and also in the private ward of the same hospital. In that way social and economic factors that might introduce statistical bias could be eliminated. "The number of controls was arbitrary, but we wanted to be sure that it was big enough to eliminate any questions," Herbst said.

A questionnaire was then designed for the thirty-two controls. There were seven significant areas of interest: the mother's age when she delivered, whether she smoked at least ten cigarettes daily during pregnancy, whether there was bleeding during pregnancy, whether there was any prior pregnancy loss, whether estrogens were taken during pregnancy, whether there was breast-feeding, and whether there had been any intrauterine X-ray exposure during pregnancy.

There were other questions as well, which could appear to be chatty and anecdotal but which in retrospect provide a clue as to the precision with which this initial study was conducted. These extra questions elicited information about birth weight, age when menstruation began, complications and outcome of pregnancy, other medicines taken during pregnancy, childhood diseases of mothers and patients, history of tonsillectomy, any substances taken during childhood, household pets, noteworthy illnesses, cosmetics used by mothers and patients, cigarette smoking by patients, alcohol use by parents, occupation and education of parents.

Household pets? Use of cosmetics? "We wanted to test what might be associated with this unusual phenomenon," Herbst said. "We were being very exhaustive purposefully to really be certain that we weren't focusing on trying to prove that something was true, but rather testing whether it was an association ... When you design a questionnaire, you've got to be careful not to design it in a way to provoke the response you *may* be looking for."

The conclusions were historic and, after their 1971 publication, irrefutable: Seven of the eight mothers whose daughters had later developed clear-cell adenocarcinoma of the vagina had taken DES during pregnancy; not one of the thirty-two controls had been so exposed. All of the women who took DES started it in the first three months of pregnancy, and they had all taken DES because of bleeding during the pregnancy.

What about the one woman who developed vaginal cancer whose mother had apparently *not* taken DES? Since clear-cell adenocarcinoma had been known to develop in older women before the synthesis of DES, the investigators believed that factors other than maternal stilbestrol ingestion appeared to be operative in its development.

Four of the eight women with vaginal cancer had sisters who had also been exposed to DES during their mothers' pregnancies, but those four women did not develop cancer. Why? The paper suggested that DES may have acted as some kind of an "initiator" of cancer, which was fully stimulated later on by certain chemical changes in the body during puberty.

What was the risk of a DES daughter getting this vaginal cancer? The numbers in the study indicated the risk was small, although the paper did not provide an exact figure. But, the report stated, the presence of adenosis, the benign cellular formation in the vagina "may be a predisposing condition."

Other people in the medical community originally speculated that the cancer risk for DES daughters might be as high as 4 in 1,000, a rate that would indicate a real epidemic. Very soon afterward, however, the cancer rate was seen as being no greater than 1.4 people in every 1,000. But since the exact number of exposed people was and is unknown, and nothing is more frightening in American health care than cancer, genuine dread was felt in many households all across the country. That dread focused at the time only on cancer, because none of the other reproductive tract problems in both sons and daughters, or health problems among mothers, was known. Concern about those problems would come later.

Once the data had been prepared, analyzed, and double-checked, the question was, what to do with it? The Herbst, Ulfelder, and Poskanzer study had clearly articulated a national medical emergency: DES had now been associated with a rare form of vaginal cancer in women, and it was still on pharmacy shelves around the country, was still being prescribed by doctors in all fifty states.

Ulfelder showed the findings to a consultant to the U.S. Surgeon

General for population affairs and was astonished at his lack of concern. The other side of that bitter coin is that while statistically incontrovertible data existed showing the association between DES use during pregnancy and vaginal cancer years later in daughters, a key federal consultant shrugged it off.

The historic paper was published in the April 22, 1971, issue of the *New England Journal of Medicine*. An editorial in the same edition called it "an original publication of great scientific importance and serious social implications." The paper's findings, the editorial said, supplied new information about the mechanism of tumor growth and added "a new dimension to the whole matter of what drugs are safe or unsafe to administer to pregnant women . . . until [the cell mechanism of adenocarcinoma] has been established, it seems prudent for physicians to use caution in prescribing estrogenic substances during pregnancy. Indeed, physicians must think more seriously before administering any drug to a pregnant woman."

The article and the editorial were picked up and synthesized, synopsized, and republished in newspapers, magazines, and television and radio newscasts all around the country. In New York State, Peter Greenwald, M.D. (director of the Cancer Control Bureau of the state's Department of Health), checked the records of the state's cancer registry for cases of clear-cell adenocarcinoma. There had been five cases recently, all in women born between 1951 and 1953, all to mothers who had taken DES during pregnancy. Three of the five girls had died.

Greenwald's findings in New York confirmed the Boston results, providing what scientists regard as independent corroboration that brings an observation beyond the realm of chance and into the realm of certainty. His findings were published in the August 12, 1971, issue of the *New England Journal of Medicine*. An editorial in the same issue stated that the cluster of cases later associated with DES "exceeds the number of cases in the entire world literature for a tumor of this type in girls born before 1945."

Before his findings were published, Greenwald sent them to New York State Commissioner of Health Hollis Ingraham, who, in June 1971, sent an urgent "Dear Doctor" letter to the more than 37,000 physicians in New York State, stating that "synthetic estrogens are contraindicated in pregnancy." Ingraham also sent a letter to the FDA, urging it to ban DES and other synthetic estrogens from use in pregnancy because of the Herbst and Greenwald reports.

The FDA took no action. The Herbst report had come out in April, the Ingraham letter had come out in June, the Greenwald report had come out in August, but the FDA took no action until Congressman L. H. Fountain called for public hearings on the subject to begin November 11, 1971. Fountain, a South Carolina congressman, had held other hearings on the controversy surrounding the use of DES as an animal growth stimulant.

On November 9, 1971, the FDA placed a notice in the Federal Register, the official daily record of government actions, announcing that DES was contraindicated for use during pregnancy. The notice was published on November 10, the day before the hearings began.

Congressman Fountain and his staff questioned FDA Commissioner Charles Edwards on why the federal watchdog agency had taken no action once it had been notified of the Herbst report, the Greenwald report, or the Ingraham letter. Agency representatives testified that they had been researching the issue and consulting with authorities around the country, but when pressed, they could produce no documentation to substantiate their position. FDA Commissioner Edwards said he thought that Ingraham's letter had been "premature . . . Not that his actions are necessarily wrong, but I think he could well have studied it a little more than he did."

Between the publication date of the Herbst report and the FDA's ban on DES use for pregnancy, an estimated twenty thousand American women took DES to prevent miscarriages, according to Barbara Seaman, coauthor of the authoritative book *Women and the Crisis in Sex Hormones*.

The congressional staff and the FDA representatives then got into a complex argument over whether DES was actually effective, and whether its perceived effectiveness warranted keeping it on the market even after the Herbst and Greenwald studies. The FDA said it did. Henry Simmons, director of the FDA's Bureau of Drugs, testified that although evidence of the effectiveness of DES did not exist, the FDA did not have evidence of its ineffectiveness. He mentioned the 1968 finding of the National Academy of Sciences that DES had been found to be "possibly effective," and added, "I suspect that some women could feel the risk of use of such drugs was warranted, with the hope of producing a live child, even though that live child, now on present evidence, may have the possibility of producing another action" that might be harmful, such as cancer.

Committee staff physician Delphis Goldman, M.D., was conducting the question at this point, and he told Simmons: "What you are doing is weighing the possibility, without any evidence of effectiveness, that a drug may be effective and may be helpful to that woman, against the possibility that she may deliver a daughter who will develop cancer of the vagina."

If DES had not been associated with cancer at all, or had been associated with a common form of cancer that would not strike even the most punctilious of researchers as unusual, would anyone now know about all the problems linked to it?

Arthur L. Herbst, M.D., said in an interview that "DES-related problems would have shown up, [although perhaps] not as quickly or as focused or in as short a period of time. The [noncancerous] changes are sufficiently unusual so that somebody would have said, 'This just *looks* funny, I wonder what's going on.'"

Arthur Herbst had two mentors as a medical student and young staff physician at Harvard and Massachusetts General Hospital: Howard Ulfelder and George Van Siclen Smith. It was with Ulfelder and others that he put together the data showing that DES was the world's first transplacental carcinogen; it was to his other mentor, George Smith, that he went seeking information and medical records of the women who had taken it during pregnancy.

"Yes, I did have anomalous feelings about it," Herbst said. "I feel great warmth for them. George and Olive Smith are honest scientists, great humanitarians, and first-class people. But all of us in medicine feel if you're dealing in knowledge, then that's what you're in the business for, and this was obviously a problem. They were concerned, but they made all their research files available to me so we could chase down some of these young ladies and make our first studies of what other changes they had had."

"Arthur Herbst was a good friend; he had trained under me," George Smith said. "He came out here and said, 'What do you think?' We told him to tell the truth. He didn't want to get us mixed up in something he thought might get us into trouble. We were surprised, we felt awful," Smith said.

"We were horrified," Olive Smith said, "when Herbst showed us their results. It was absolute horror. Our reaction was, in trying to help we had done a terrible thing. We quoted our then six-year-old grandson after he had accidentally broken his father's slide projector: 'Even when I try to do good I do bad.' After all our years of trying to help people . . . But we know now we didn't do bad—it was absolutely sound. This was given to millions of women throughout the world from 1948 to 1971. I can't believe obstetricians would use it if it didn't work. It was not a wonder drug, we had lots of failures . . ."

The Smiths say their work has been distorted by both the lay press and by doctors themselves.

These last few years have been difficult for the Smiths, staining what they had thought would be a trouble-free retirement when they would bask in the glow of the work they had done in bringing a precise knowledge of endocrinology to bear on how the body works during pregnancy. Instead they have had a succession of drug company lawyers troop down to their basement to gather material from their files of women treated with DES, for use in defending the companies against lawsuits brought by people exposed to DES.

George Smith retired from active practice several years ago when he felt he was no longer physically up to its demands and now works on his memoirs, as well as consulting with former patients who visit their home. When people want medical records, the Smiths ask them to send stamped return envelopes, because their funds are limited. "I saw many DES girls in my office and none of them had clear-cell or adenosis," George Smith said. The Smiths feel that their work and their theory will be vindicated in the years to come and that DES will be returned to the medical list of approved drugs for use in certain pregnancies.

"The kind of work George and I were doing is almost getting nonallowed," Olive Smith said, "—experimenting on humans. Our whole idea was to find out how things work." And, she said, since there was no animal model that completely duplicated the human response, work on humans was essential. "It's been an upsetting experience because it's been so distorted," she repeated. "We picked the hard way, we wanted to help—"

"We wanted to save babies," George Smith bellowed, concluding her thought.

Now they have a coterie of close friends and former colleagues who lend support and encouragement. The George Van Siclen Smith and Olive Watkins Smith Fund for Reproductive Endocrinology has been established in their honor at Brigham and Women's Hospital, a teaching affiliate of the Harvard Medical School.

Joanne Smith died on November 4, 1976, at the age of twenty-seven. The cause of her death was associated with the vaginal cancer that had spread to her lungs. She weighed sixty-three pounds. In the last six years of her life she had undergone a partial vaginectomy, radiation therapy five times a week for a recurrence of vaginal cancer, radium implants, and removal of her colon and bladder.

A doctor who examined Joanne right before her vaginectomy told her parents that she was the thirty-third such known case in America.

Doris M. Smith, Joanne's mother, had had one tubal pregnancy in 1948 and was told she might never have any children at all. In early 1949 Doris became pregnant again, and although her physician did not believe it was a tubal pregnancy, he sent her to a hospital during the third month of the pregnancy. Throughout the spring and summer of 1949 Mrs. Smith (then a housewife in Westfield, New Jersey) took DES during her pregnancy with Joanne. Mrs. Smith's medical records prove it. "I don't recall taking DES, but after Joanne became ill, we saw the doctor's records, and the records said 'stilbestrol.'"

"I was just back from the war, making $2,240 a year as a rookie on the Westfield police force," John B. Smith said. "I thought that was good money [about $43 a week], because eighteen-dollar-a-week jobs were pretty common too. We were a young couple struggling along, and those were different times. I truthfully feel that back in those days doctors were looked on almost as minor gods. Did a doctor want you to take a bath in the lake? You did it, you had faith."

Late in 1970, during her second year of college, Joanne needed a blood test so she could get a marriage license. Her father told her to get a complete physical at the same time, "just as a convenience," he said. The internist saw something he didn't like and referred her to a DES specialist, just as word of cancer problems associated with DES was beginning to filter out. Her November 1970 wedding was postponed for two months while she recovered from the partial hysterectomy that was performed. She was twenty-one years old.

"They thought they'd gotten it all," John Smith said. "Funny thing, a year earlier she'd had her appendix taken out and no one had spotted anything."

After her marriage Joanne and her husband contacted adoption agencies, since they could not have children of their own. They were turned down. Her mother recalls that the reason given was the past existence of cancer. "We know now that this was the right decision of the adoption agencies, but at the time, when we all hoped there would be no recurrence of the cancer, it seemed unfair. Because of DES Joanne was denied the privilege of being a mother, which is an important part of a woman's life," Mrs. Smith wrote me.

Four years after Joanne's hysterectomy the cancer recurred, and she began radiation treatment five times a week. In 1975 her colon and bladder were removed, and by 1976 the cancer had spread to her lungs.

"It was and is a time bomb," Doris Smith now says quietly. "We were told there was a ninety-nine percent chance everything would be fine, but after 1974 it was awful."

On her deathbed, Joanne, a religious woman who had gone to a Christian college, looked up at her father and said, "The suffering I've gone through is nothing compared to what Jesus did for me."

She was buried in a closed casket on her sister Patti's birthday, November 8, 1976.

A lawsuit against several drug companies was settled out of court in the late 1970s for thirty thousand dollars, Mrs. Smith said. In such settlements, liability is never admitted. Doris Smith said she had no idea which company made the DES she took, only that the prescription for it was listed on her medical records.

Joanne's sister, Patti Smith Mazzarelle, a San Diego, California, resident with two school-age children, is still disturbed by Joanne's death. I had first spoken with her in the summer of 1981 in her home, where new kitchen cabinets were sitting on the floor waiting to be installed and finished. She was then working as a foster parent for local welfare agencies. She was also active in the area DES Action chapter.

"Watching your sister die is not easy. I was with her the last six weeks, giving her morphine injections to ease the pain. I didn't cry until it was all over. It's real hard being separated from her. I miss her more *now*," she said. She spoke quickly and nervously and with great force, animation, and love for her sister, whose cheerful smile comes through the color snapshots Patti keeps like a testimonial. "For the first two years after her death I sat in a rocker and rocked. I decided to see a psychiatrist. I'm DES-exposed too, and one day my son asked me, 'If you're a DES daughter, am I a DES son?' "

When I called back as I was writing this chapter, Patti Mazzarelle said in a subdued voice: "The fifth anniversary of my sister's death was in November, and I couldn't handle it anymore. I had a nervous breakdown, a term the doctors used. I was in a mental hospital for a week. I was totally unable to function. A psychiatrist discussed my foster-care work with me and said I had lost my sister and was trying to replace her with each new baby. I don't know if I buy that, but he's supposed to know more about these things than I am."

She has given up her foster-care work and also cut down on her volunteer work with DES Action because it put too great a strain on her, she said.

Her father, on the phone from the mobile home park he and Doris now manage, acknowledged the difficulty his daughter was having: "I would have hoped with time she would have gotten over it. For some reason she has trouble coping. It's very hard for us as parents to see her like that." Patti's mother wonders if "she'd be having these problems today if she hadn't been with me while we cared for Joanne at home for the last six weeks of here life. But I don't know if I could have gotten through it without her." For the parents, as Doris Smith says, "there are so many memories. Joanne was reserved, and studied hard, and was never any trouble to us. She was a loving and caring person."

John Smith recalled fondly: "Once in a while we'll be riding along in a car and see something nice and say, 'Gee, I'll bet Joanne—,' and then you realize she's not here anymore. I grew up on a big old dairy farm; you saw death and sickness as a part of life. I could accept this in a way, but it was hard for me to see what my wife and kids were going through. I became very depressed—I had to take medication. This can really upset you."

Doris, like her husband a calm and thoughtful and decent person, said she does not feel guilty about taking DES during pregnancy because, "the doctor said it would help. No one said, if you take it such and so will happen, nobody knew about the future. But not a day goes by that we don't think of her," Doris Smith told me. "She suffered so much that death was a blessing." She says she does not feel guilt, "except way back in the corner of my mind." But speaking really for both of them, her husband put in gently, "You do have your quiet moments, though."

The stories of cancer caused by or associated with DES usage during pregnancy have horrified mothers, daughters, sons, and fathers in this country for more than a decade. It was the first aspect of the DES story to break and the one to strike more terror into the hearts of more households than anything else associated with this bitter pill. For the millions of DES-exposed people who have *not* gotten cancer, the relief is palpable, even though that relief is tempered by a lack of information as to what will happen in the future.

As of June 1, 1980, 429 cases had been listed with the Registry for Research on Hormonal Transplacental Carcinogenesis, which was set up specifically by Arthur L. Herbst, M.D., and others to monitor all the reported cases. It is based in Chicago. According to the Registry, mothers whose daughters got cancer took as little as one milligram a day of DES or as much as 300 milligrams daily. Over the course of their pregnancies the mothers of daughters with cancer took as little as 131 milligrams and as much as 21,400 milligrams. A seven-year-old girl got cancer; so did a thirty-one-year-old woman. Most of the cancer cases occurred when the young women were between the ages of fourteen and twenty-four. In 80 percent of the cases the mothers of the cancer patients had begun DES treatment in the first 12 weeks of pregnancy.

In one study of 400 women with clear-cell adenocarcinoma, there were 79 deaths, 12 women living with the disease, 12 women who had had a recurrence and were living and well, and 297 women who had had the disease once and were living and well.

In a 1981 textbook on DES, *Developmental Effects of Diethylstilbestrol (DES) in Pregnancy*, edited by Herbst and Howard A. Bern, Ph.D. (professor of zoology and research endocrinologist at the University of California at Berkeley), there is a chart listing the number of clear-cell adenocarcinoma cases with confirmed DES exposure on a state-by-state basis. Its simple numerical listing goes a long way toward showing the widespread use of DES throughout the United States and disproving the idea that it was primarily used in the Northeast. In California, the nation's largest state, there were 34 cases; in Alaska, the smallest state in the country, there were 2 cases. New York had 25, Washington State had 6, Texas had 5, West Virginia had 2, Massachusetts had 17, Pennsylvania had 14, Oregon had 2, and Maine had 4.

The Registry also has 4 DES-positive cases from Canada, 4 from Australia, 3 from France, 2 from Great Britain, and one each from Mexico, Belgium, Holland, Czechoslovakia, and the Ivory Coast of Africa—statistics that graphically illustrate the worldwide nature of the DES phenomenon.

Arthur L. Herbst, M.D., speculated later in the text that since adenocarcinoma of the vagina and cervix had been previously seen in older women, there might be another recurrence of adenocarcinoma cases when exposed women get older.

In a southern city I was introduced to a woman whose daughter-in-law had documented DES exposure and had recently died from clear-cell adenocarcinoma. The woman's son and the deceased young woman had been childhood sweethearts. Their long-planned marriage had been put off, and at times canceled, because the girl believed she would "not last long," the mother-in-law told me.

The young woman had had cysts on her vagina and medical records showing she had been DES-exposed, but despite the warning signs, she had often refused medical treatment or mental-health therapy, believing it was hopeless. During the last year of her life she had completely refused medical care and had died in November 1980. Now, the mother said, her son, who lives at home, drinks six beers a night and smokes marijuana incessantly. "One night I heard him up at four in the morning. Since I couldn't sleep either, I went down to his room and said I didn't know why I was having trouble sleeping. My son said, 'Well, I know why I can't sleep—it's because I always see her face when I shut my eyes.' "

Mary Beth Roth is twenty-eight years old and has had confirmed DES exposure, but the cancer that caused the surgical removal of both ovaries, both fallopian tubes, and her uterus was *not* adenocarcinoma. It is called serous papillary tumors of low malignant potential. There has never been a connection made between this kind of ovarian cancer in humans and *in utero* exposure to DES.

Ovarian cancer in general is now on the increase, and Mary Beth Roth is younger than most women who get this kind of cancer, who are usually in their fifties. According to the American Cancer Society, 18,-000 cases of ovarian cancer will be seen this year, including 11,000 cases that will result in death.

DES is associated with cancerous development in the vagina, cervix, and endometrium. Those areas are free of disease in Mary Beth Roth. The areas that had deposits of malignant cells were both ovaries, one fallopian tube, and broad ligaments. Surgery removed bilateral masses in both ovaries and malignant tumors in both fallopian tubes—areas that have not been associated with DES-type cancers.

A 1982 medical study found an unusually high incidence of a relatively rare, benign ovarian tumor in three of 350 DES daughters examined at the University of North Carolina in Chapel Hill. Physicians Grant Schmidt and Wesley C. Fowler, Jr. stated in their *Gynecologic Oncology* article that while a cause-and-effect relationship between the tumors and DES exposure was unclear, DES daughters in their twenties and thirties should be regularly examined as a precaution against the development of the rare, though benign, ovarian tumor, as well as for other DES-related problems.

Regarding a potentially dangerous type of tumor of borderline malignancy found in one DES woman, they stated: "Until more information is available on the natural history of the tumors classified as borderline malignant, removal of the pelvic organs once reproductive functions have been completed is suggested." (The pelvic organs include the uterus, the fallopian tubes, and the ovaries.)

A study in the September 10, 1977, issue of *Lancet*, however, made a tentative connection between DES use during menopause and an increased risk of ovarian cancer. The letter—called a "Preliminary Communication," by American researchers Robert Hoover, Laman A. Gray, Sr., and Joseph F. Fraumeni, Jr.—looked at 908 women who had used Premarin, a form of estrogen, for menopausal symptoms. In that group there were 8 cases of ovarian cancer, a risk two or three times greater than expected. The authors wrote that "the excess risk of ovarian cancer in this group occurred primarily among 21 women who had also used stilbestrol (diethylstilbestrol)."

The focus on the relationship between cancer and DES daughters has raised questions about an increased rise of cancer in the women who took the drug. The informal study published in *Lancet* suggests that DES mothers may be more susceptible to ovarian cancer. In 1978 a study from the University of Chicago addressed the same issue. Published in the April 6, 1978, issue of the *New England Journal of Medicine*, it was a twenty-five-year follow-up of 693 women in the original Dieckmann study who had been given DES and 668 who had not received it. Of those given the drug, 32 (or 4.6 percent) had breast cancer, compared to 21 (or 3.1 percent) of the controls. The authors, headed by Marluce Bibbo, M.D., stated that the difference was "not statistically significant."

There was also a slightly higher incidence of other kinds of cancer for DES women in that study. Four had ovarian cancer (compared to one of the controls), 2 had colon cancer (compared to one of the controls), 7 had cervical cancer (compared to 3 unexposed women who had it), and there were 18 cancers of other types (undescribed) for the DES women, compared to 15 for the unexposed.

All told, 66 DES women (or 9.5 percent) had gotten cancer of some type, compared to 46 women (or 6.9 percent) of the unexposed. The authors of the study concluded that these were not significant differences.

The incidence of breast cancer in DES mothers was the second major cancer issue to surface in the DES phenomenon. In 1977 Sidney Wolfe, M.D., director of the Health Research Group, used the federal Freedom of Information Act to obtain the preliminary data from the University of Chicago study. Using an analytical method that focused on the ages of the DES mothers, Wolfe concluded that they were indeed at a far greater risk of getting breast cancer at an earlier age than unexposed women, a far greater risk of dying from that breast cancer, and that the difference in risk was statistically significant. His analysis was double-checked and ratified by Food and Drug Administration statistician Adrian Gross and was in part responsible for an FDA advisory on the subject sent to physicians in the spring of 1978.

Wolfe's analysis, and the widespread concern it generated among the public, led to several articles in medical journals supporting the Chicago position—that the numerical increase was not statistically significant—as well as at least one medical article supporting Wolfe, who has not backed off from his analysis and maintains that the breast cancer risks for mothers is significant.

The Herbst-Bern textbook cites these figures on the subject, based on women from the Dieckmann study: there were 14 DES mothers between the ages of forty and forty-nine with breast cancer, compared to 7 unexposed women in the same age group with breast cancer. There were 15 DES mothers over fifty with breast cancer, compared to 12 unexposed women over fifty. Regarding death due to breast cancer, 15 DES mothers had died, compared to 6 unexposed mothers. When deaths from breast cancer and other cancers were all factored together, 27 DES mothers had died, compared to 15 unexposed mothers.

The paper (by Marian M. Hubby, Ph.D., William M. Haenszel, Dr. P.H., and Herbst) quoted in the textbook maintained the earlier position that the figures did not show a statistical difference but added:

> The earlier appearance of breast cancer cases among exposed women prior to age 50 (17 cases of breast cancer among the exposed compared to 9 among controls) merits attention. The possibility that a DES-effect might be concentrated in the premenopausal ages following administration of the drug deserves investigation. However, since chance variation cannot be ruled out as the explanation for the group difference in overall number of breast cancers, all comparisons of subgroups of mothers must be cautiously interpreted and treated with reserve.

The paper concluded:

> The data available on the long-term effect on mothers of DES taken during pregnancy do not indicate an adverse effect on the mothers' health. An earlier occurrence of breast cancer among those exposed to DES, although not statistically significant, has raised concerns about a possible DES effect and should be investigated in other groups of exposed women if possible. The medical management of DES-exposed mothers at present requires no special diagnostic test such as mammography ... Regular physical and breast examination is important for women exposed to DES, as it is for all women in this age group.

Anecdotally, some DES mothers have complained of thyroid problems and other problems related to endocrine function, but as yet there are no definitive studies on this. Given the extraordinary power of DES and its known ability to influence the body's functions down to the tiniest stromal layer, further discoveries of abnormal activities may yet be made.

That is why it is just as crucial for mothers to find out for their own sakes if they took DES as well as for the sake of their children. At the same time, researchers also point out that the mothers who took DES are only now entering menopause, and that types of cancer occurring later in life in the general population may appear more frequently with them than with nonexposed women.

Discussions of cancer and DES primarily focus on the young women, many of them teenagers, who have had clear-cell adenocarcinoma. I met a nurse who was able to place the subject in a humane, compassionate framework. She is the head nurse in the gynecological oncology section of a major teaching hospital on the east coast. A large, affable woman who radiates warmth and sympathy and confidence, she is the kind of person you'd want near you if you were sick. In her career she has seen about ten DES daughters who have required "surgical intervention," young women between the ages of fourteen and twenty-six who needed vaginectomies and hysterectomies because of adenocarcinoma. She had even attended one woman in the late 1970s who delivered a baby and then had surgery performed.

"They need a lot of support, a lot of time and understanding. There's more to it than just surgery. Ninety-nine percent of them have never been in hospitals before, now they come in and they're told, 'hysterectomy, radical vaginectomy.' They're told their vagina will be removed; they're young, just kids, it's hard for them to handle. A new vagina can be constructed from a skin graft, but the sensitivity varies. One patient almost refused the surgery because of the vaginectomy. She focused on the scar. She was angry, angry, angry. She wanted no memory of her problems."

On the walls of the nurse's office are color pictures of some of her patients, the faces of women once again healthy, back in their own worlds, on their front lawns, grinning up into the flash, sending their photos back to the nurses who were there "24 hours a day" when they went through the traumatic experiences that literally should never have happened.

"It's not the same thing as a mastectomy. If you keep talking about it like a cheerleader, it can get to you. But peer counseling can help, show they're not alone. The thing with DES patients is, we're getting strong, young healthy women—with cancer. They sometimes have a tremendous body-image problem. One of them had worked so hard on getting a beautiful body, and now it would be marred by a scar. The scars go away better with a younger person, but still . . .

"If the patient is too young, under eighteen, an explanation of the surgery is given in front of her parent or guardian. The mothers sometimes have guilt—they took the pills. The fathers are heartbroken, because it's Daddy's little girl, but often they are very supportive to both the mother and the daughter. Afterward the parents can sometimes smother, they become too overprotective; others are very supportive. As for their records [showing DES exposure], sometimes it's almost like someone got there before them."

A nurse sees things doctors may miss or not focus on: "You come back from the surgery and you're sick. There's a tube in your nose, a catheter in your side. What twenty-one-year-old wants to go home with a bag on her leg? One patient called it a 'pee bag.' There can be complications afterward, especially cramping, and skin irritation. It's like a sorority or club, and after a certain point it can get to them. They feel labeled 'DES.' Do people love them more because they've had this? Will men take advantage of them because they can't get pregnant? Will men want to test out an artificial vagina? How do they stop feeling sorry for themselves?"

She remembers two patients in particular. "One had her uterus removed, a partial vaginectomy, her ovaries were left in. She recently stopped by—she was happier than before, feeling good, she'd had a good summer. Who knows in two or three years if her anger will be stirred up again? Another woman, 'Mary,' did well after surgery, but she still has difficulty with the labeling of the disease. She's met a fellow, likes him a lot, but she's still questioning, why is he so fond of her? Could someone else love her?"

But the patients are not the only ones troubled by the problem. For nurses in her cancer ward, she said, it is sometimes difficult, more than they anticipate. "The thing with DES is that the patients are the same age as many of the nurses. But we are a part of their family. We're a part of their lives that will be forever remembered. Whether skilled nursing carried them along to die, or to health, it carried them along."

8

PREMATURE BIRTHS

In the anxiety over the relationship between DES and cancer that began in 1971, little attention was devoted to other aspects of DES exposure. But as the decade closed, a wide variety of other medical problems experienced by both daughters and sons of DES mothers began bubbling to the surface in medical journals around the country.

The most agreed-upon aspect of DES exposure in daughters is that they are more likely to have premature babies than nonexposed women. The risk for this varies, depending on the study, but DES daughters were nearly two or three times more likely to have a premature baby than nonexposed women. The reasons for the increased risk of premature birth have not yet been fully documented.

The normal length of pregnancy is thirty-eight to forty weeks, and any child born earlier than that is regarded as premature. A baby born at or before the twenty-sixth week of pregnancy is usually given a very slim chance of survival; the body, especially the lungs, will not be developed enough to survive outside the intrauterine environment. Many premature babies do survive with no damage, but their health is often dependent on getting immediate intensive medical attention. But there can be serious problems in store for a premature infant, including mild to severe learning disabilities, mental retardation, neuromuscular problems (difficulties in walking and talking), damage to sensory organs such as the ears and eyes, a susceptibility to infectious diseases, slow physical and emotional development. One physician who has delivered thousands of babies said, "Prematurity can be devastating."

During the 1970s hundreds of thousands of women of childbearing age learned that they were DES-exposed and were examined for possible vaginal cancer. But none of those women, knowing they were DES-exposed, also knew that when they got pregnant they would be at a higher risk for a premature baby than other women.

Susan Elliott, for example, knew she was a DES daughter, but in 1979 she had no knowledge of the risk of premature delivery. Three days after she returned home to Washington, D.C., from a cruise through the Gulf of Alaska, she went into premature labor.

"There had been no signs of prematurity. My water broke in the middle of the night, so I went to the hospital the next morning. Almost as soon as I arrived I went into premature labor. There was a placental separation, which means the baby's blood supply was being cut off. I was expelling blood clots the size of baseballs, and the fetal monitor showed that the baby's heart was beginning to falter. But my doctor was able to deliver Tara safely by Caesarean section—she takes pride in the fact that she had Tara out of me within four minutes after they got me to the operating room," she said. "If this had happened while I was on the cruise ship, just three days earlier, with the little medical equipment they had there, the baby would have died and I could have died too. Even if the placental separation had happened at home, the baby probably would have been dead within fifteen minutes because of a lack of oxygen."

Born in 1948 in Palm Springs, California, Susan Elliott is currently assistant director of the Federal Trade Commission. She had known she was DES-exposed since 1971, when she was examined by a leading DES researcher. She had been told she had adenosis, a cervical collar, and bumps and ridges on the vaginal wall. But she had not received any warning about possible prematurity during pregnancy, because no one knew anything about that problem then. Later studies would suggest an association between cervical ridges and premature births.

She got pregnant again and in March of 1981 had a second child, who was also premature, one month early. "After each pregnancy I had atypical cells around the cervix. I had a lot of anxiety—what did this mean? Before I could find out, the condition went away."

As an attorney she is intellectually intrigued by her DES experience. "It's a fascinating question, really. When do you put new drugs on the market?" As a woman and a mother she has had to do some hard thinking. "I cast no blame whatsoever on my parents, or any of the physicians who examined me early on," Susan Elliott said. "I'm not bitter, I don't blame anyone, I've had my two kids."

✳ ✳ ✳

In 1980 the first of a series of medical papers was published detailing the noncancerous impact of DES exposure before birth. In the February 1980 issue of the *Journal of Reproductive Medicine,* Arthur L. Herbst, M.D., Marian M. Hubby, Ph.D., Richard R. Blough, M.S., and Freidoon Azizi, M.D., published a paper titled "A Comparison of Pregnancy Experience in DES-Exposed and DES-Unexposed Daughters." (Herbst, who had been at Massachusetts General Hospital at the time he coauthored the famous 1971 DES/cancer paper, had gone to Chicago in 1976.)

The paper compared the reproductive histories of 226 DES-exposed daughters with those of 203 unexposed women. The mothers of the women in both groups had been a part of the original Dieckmann study in the 1950s. The summary stated: "Premature live birth was experienced by 22% of the exposed but only 7% of the unexposed" meaning that DES daughters were more than three times likely to have a premature live birth than nonexposed women. "The reason for the higher incidence of prematurity . . . among the DES-exposed is not clear." The authors speculated, drawing on other reports, that the presence of the cervicovaginal ridges might play a part, as might such structural abnormalities as a T-shaped or otherwise misshapen uterus, or a shortened or weaker cervix.

One month later, in March 1980, another major paper was issued. This one represented the latest findings of the federally funded DESAD (DES/Adenosis) project. The DESAD project had been established as part of the federal government's effort to determine on a nationwide basis what had happened medically as a result of DES usage during pregnancy. Published in the *New England Journal of Medicine,* the article concluded that DES daughters in their study were at a somewhat greater risk for prematurity than nonexposed women, but that the actual risk was considerably less than Herbst had found.

In this DESAD paper the unfavorable reproductive experiences of 220 DES daughters from around the country were compared to the reproductive experiences of 224 nonexposed women. Considering the subject of prematurity, the authors found that 17 of the DES daughters (or 7.7 percent) had had premature births, compared to 10 (or 4.5 percent) of the nonexposed women. This study calculated the risk factor to be 1.71, meaning that a DES daughter was nearly twice as likely to be at risk for a premature baby as an unexposed daughter.

The study (whose lead author was Ann B. Barnes, M.D.) presented an analysis of the amounts of DES taken by pregnant mothers and the incidence of premature births in their daughters. "Women who gave birth prematurely had been exposed *in utero* to a higher dose of DES, administered earlier in pregnancy and for a longer duration than did those who did not have this outcome."

Looking at 12 DES women who had had premature births, the study showed that their mothers had taken a total of 3,490 milligrams of DES, starting at the 84th day of pregnancy and continuing for 162 days more. By contrast, mothers of DES women in the study who had not had a premature birth had taken a total of 2,415 milligrams, starting at the 97th day and continuing for 130 days. "The strongest dose-response relation was found for premature births," the paper stated. "Women who gave birth prematurely had been exposed *in utero* to a higher dose of DES, administered earlier in pregnancy and for a longer duration than those who did not have this outcome."

The paper also took a look at the relationship, if any, between premature births and structural anomalies of the reproductive system. "We could detect no difference in outcome of pregnancy in this study between DES-exposed women with and without structural anomalies; however, the number with anomalies is small (only 36) . . . The apparent risk in both groups with and without structural anomalies is still higher than that in the controls; . . . Current epidemiologic data do not indicate a particular biologic mechanism."

The paper does speculate, however, on possible factors affecting women who have experienced premature births and miscarriages. "The miscarriages and premature births seen to date could as likely come from sepsis [the presence in the blood or tissue of harmful microorganisms or poisons], from faulty placental attachment anywhere in the uterus, or from some collagenous [proteinlike substance in the tissue], muscular, neurologic, or hormonal incompetence of the inner cervical os [opening]. With all patients, before any therapeutic intervention is indicated, it must be clear that cervical or uterine incompetence is the cause of the disruption of pregnancy."

More than a year later, in the December 15, 1981, issue of the *American Journal of Obstetrics and Gynecology,* Arthur L. Herbst, Marian M. Hubby, Freidoon Azizi, and Michael M. Makii analyzed in part the reproductive experiences of 338 DES daughters and 298 unexposed women. All the mothers of women in the study had been given DES by William Dieckmann at the University of Chicago's Lying-In Hospital in the early 1950s, and the study was a continuation of the one they had published a year earlier.

DES daughters in the study were more than three times as likely to have a premature baby as nonexposed women. Looking at premature births only within the group, the authors discovered that 20 percent of the DES daughters had had premature births (after a pregnancy period of more than twenty-six weeks), compared to only 6 percent of the nonexposed daughters. The paper stated:

> An unfavorable pregnancy outcome is much more likely among the exposed women. Premature birth is much more common. While many of the infants survived, some were too immature for extrauterine life. Under appropriate circumstances midpregnancy losses can be effectively treated by cervical cerclage [a surgical stitch that closes the cervix and thus helps to strengthen its ability to hold the growing fetus in place] . . . This procedure is reserved for those DES-exposed women who have traditional obstetric indications for its use—a history of prior midpregnancy losses or premature dilation of the cervix in the absence of other complications.

Elsewhere in the paper the authors looked at incidence of cervicovaginal ridges, ridges on the normally smooth upper vaginal area that are more common in DES-exposed daughters. Among the DES daughters who had ridges, 43 percent had an adverse pregnancy outcome, including prematurity, while 17 percent of those without a ridge had an adverse result. "Adverse pregnancy outcome is more likely in DES-exposed subjects with cervicovaginal ridges," the authors stated.

They looked at DES daughters with vaginal epithelial changes, or changes on the cellular surface of the vagina. Of the women who had vaginal epithelial changes, 32 percent had an adverse outcome, compared to 20 percent without the changes.

The paper reported that the mean dosage of DES taken throughout their entire pregnancy by the mothers in the original 1950s study was 12,031 milligrams—the same dosage recommended by George and Olive Smith, which was also advocated by a number of drug companies (including Eli Lilly) and many physicians.

There has developed in the DES field a certain amount of intramural rivalry between people conducting DES studies as to which study most accurately reflects the risks involved for DES offspring. That rivalry has tended to confuse the public and lay press, which reads or hears that "a major study" of DES has reached a certain conclusion. It takes a while to sort out the players, but in general, the Herbst study, based on records from women only in the University of Chicago's 1950s study, deals with women who took larger doses of DES over a longer period of time than those involved in the DESAD project, which compiles information from six clinics and hospitals around the country based on the experience of people whose mothers took it in varying doses for varying lengths of time.

For example, in the 1981 Herbst paper mentioned above, the mean dosage of DES taken by mothers of women in the study was 12,031 milligrams. That study found that DES-exposed daughters faced nearly a three times greater risk of premature delivery than nonexposed women in the study. But in the 1980 DESAD study, the mean dosage of DES taken by mothers whose daughters had premature births was 3,490 milligrams, and daughters in that study were at less than a two times greater risk of prematurity.

Clearly there is an association between *in utero* DES use and a chance of premature delivery decades later by a daughter, but the precise risk depends upon a wide variety of factors, including dosage, length of time the drug was taken, health care, and medical practice.

The DES experience has been a deductive process: something is seen, and researchers spend years searching for an association between what they see and the causes. It was that way with the association between clear-cell adenocarcinoma in young women and DES use by their mothers years earlier. It will undoubtedly be that way too with the increased risk of premature births experienced by DES daughters.

During its fourth week of life a human embryo is about one-fifth of an inch long, slightly longer than a grain of rice. The cells that will develop into human organs are present but in an undifferentiated state. What will become the female reproductive tract starts from a tiny organic structure called the mesonephric ridge. From this ridge will develop the müllerian duct (first described by the early nineteenth-century German physiologist Johannes Peter Müller). The müllerian ducts will play a crucial role in the development of the fallopian tubes, uterus, and parts of the vagina.

All of this development is going on during the first few weeks of life. The embryo (it is not called a fetus until the eighth week) floats in a sea of amniotic fluid, getting maternal blood and oxygen from the placenta. In the four-week-old embryo, the neural tube, from which the central nervous system will develop, is still open.

By the fifth week the embryo, now two-fifths of an inch long, has obtained features that identify it as human—eyes, hands, and arms can be seen, as well as a vestigial tail. In the sixth week the embryo is three-fifths of an inch long, with a growing brain and discernible liver and heart. As the seventh week of gestation progresses, the embryo develops a truly recognizable human form: about one inch long—as long as a thumb joint—it has a large head and discrete arms and legs, and facial features start to become distinct. In another week, the eighth week of gestation, the mother may feel a kick from the growing fetus.

During the remainder of the first trimester, or three months, of intra-uterine life, the fetus will grow a few millimeters each day, more and more acquiring human shape and form. At the end of the first trimester the fetus will weigh about seven ounces, have a length of about six inches, and will push out against the amniotic sac. It is during the first four months of gestation that the cells of the body are multiplying, changing, evolving, and growing into the intricately complex organism known as a person. Many organs won't yet be fully formed, and their development can be influenced by outside factors.

The baby lives inside the amniotic sac, which grows inside the mother's uterus. The placenta forms a life-support system around the sac. In the placenta there is a thin membrane that separates the baby's blood from the mother's blood and screens out all large protein mole-cules or blood corpuscles that might harm the baby, since its delicate system would be unable to absorb them. Nutrients and oxygen do pass through this membrane, entering the baby's system through the umbili-cal cord, which also carries waste products and carbon dioxide away from the baby and into the mother's blood, which eliminates them.

For years it was widely believed that the placenta acted as an absolute barrier against harmful substances passing from the pregnant woman to the baby. The theory held that chemically harmful substances would "bind" to this membrane, as if a kite had gotten stuck flat against a chain link fence. Therefore, it was thought, any harmful substances that a mother ingested would be kept from the baby by means of this pla-cental barrier.

One of the first hints of the invalidity of this theory came in the 1940s when it was shown that German measles experienced early in pregnancy could cause birth defects in a child. Until then the cause-and-effect relationship between the disease and handicapped children had never been established. Another shattering proof that at least some substances crossed the placenta came in the thalidomide tragedy of the 1960s. Thalidomide was apparently the world's first drug known to cross the placenta and harm an embryo or fetus, though not kill it. Taken early in pregnancy, it crossed the placenta and stunted or stopped the development of the cells that are destined to grow into arms and legs. Thalidomide affected thousands of people; DES affected millions.

Once in the body, DES passed through the placental barrier and, for reasons not yet known, was able to affect the development of the reproductive tract of the embryo or fetus. DES is a nonsteroidal estrogen, which means it does not have the four interlocking carbon rings other natural estrogens have. That was the intent when Sir Charles Dodds worked on its structure in 1938—to simplify a compound that would imitate the actions of natural estrogens, which DES did. There is currently some speculation in the medical field that the nonsteroidal shape of DES may have something to do with its ability to affect developing cells. One theory is that this shape may make it harder for the liver to metabolize DES, so that DES stays in the body for a longer time.

Once it passes the placental barrier, DES acts on the multiplying and changing cells of what will become the reproductive system in ways that are still unclear. Because there are structural differences in the cervix, uterus, and vagina of some DES daughters, it may be that DES acts directly on those cells to change their shape. Or perhaps it acts on natural chemicals in the body, which affect the growing cells.

Clear-cell adenocarcinoma may be triggered years later by the chemical changes brought on by menarche. That possibility led Arthur L. Herbst and others to express concern about cancer development in DES daughters when they go through menopause—another time the body goes through a great many hormonal changes.

One physician, who knows he is among a minority of doctors who believe that DES worked for a small select group of women, is also keenly aware of the problems DES-exposed people are having. This is the lay language he used to describe the route that DES took when swallowed, pill by pill, by millions of American women: "Look at the travels of this goddamn DES. It goes in your mouth and gets eaten up by salivary enzymes, down your esophagus, into your gut, where it's sprayed with acid and gastric juices. From the gut to the intestines to the liver, where it's metabolized as much as the liver can do, out into the circulation system, through the aorta and arteries to the uterus, then through the uterine cavity to the placenta, across the placenta barrier to the fetus. Sometime during that period the genital and reproductive tracts are developing—the exact moments aren't fixed. An individual's own biochemistry will vary for each person, so the impact will be different for each person, but during that period there's a window open providing access to the developing genital tract. You know," he said, "that there are bound to be biological variations."

With regard to the premature birth problems of women exposed to DES *in utero*, who may have had their reproductive systems changed or affected by the drug, some people have speculated that DES affects the ability of the uterus to hold onto the placenta—a possibility that is consistent with other pregnancy problems, including miscarriages. Perhaps it affects the epithelial (surface) cells in a woman's reproductive tract, or perhaps it affects the stromal (underlying) cells in the same region.

A small study from San Diego also drew attention to the increased risk of premature births in DES-exposed women. It was published in the July 1980 issue of *Obstetrics and Gynecology* and had as its principle author Larry Cousins, M.D., a staff member at the University of California's San Diego Medical Center. In that study, which relied on mailed questionnaires, there were 20 births among 71 DES-exposed women, and 8 of the 20 births—or 40 percent—were premature. By comparison, there were 69 nonexposed women, and there were no premature births among the 28 unexposed women who had children. Five of the 8 DES daughters who delivered prematurely had anatomical changes, including adenosis, cervical ridges, and a cockscomb cervix (a ridge of vaginal tissue extending around the top of the cervix).

The report stated: "Given the common müllerian duct origin of the upper vagina, cervix, uterus, and oviducts, it is not unreasonable to assume that DES-related gross changes of the cervix and vagina may also be associated with developmental anomalies of the upper genital tract . . . It is conceivable that hormonal exposure during embryogenesis [the period when the embryo is developing], which is known to produce alterations in the distribution of epithelial components, could also affect the anatomic or histological [minute tissue shape] of the underlying stroma."

"These findings," the paper concluded, "are preliminary."

The unique and unprecedented nature of the DES experience has not only prompted a series of medical studies and articles but also was the basis of the Herbst-Bern textbook dealing with DES findings in both humans and in animals. One of the chapters, written by Bern and Frank J. Talamantes, Jr., Ph.D., deals with newborn mice used as models to judge the impact of DES use in the human female. In it they state: "In neither experimental mice nor DES-exposed human offspring has sufficient attention been paid to circulatory hormone levels to be able to state whether or not other segments of the endocrine system or the neural determinants of their function have been affected. Certainly, the reproductive difficulties reported for some DES-exposed females suggest the possibility of significant endocrinologic dysfunction." The endocrine system in the human body deals with the delicate release of hormones into the circulatory system, influencing such things as general body health, sexual development, and metabolism.

Scientists in research laboratories around the world are seeking to find out how DES affects these aspects of embryonic and human life. Physicians Arthur Herbst, Ann Barnes, Larry Cousins, and others have documented the higher rate of premature births in DES-exposed women, but the reasons are still unclear. Perhaps this latest generation of research will provide some of the answers.

They might be of interest to DES daughter Carol Simpson, who also had a premature baby.

Carol Simpson's first child, Elizabeth Cady Simpson, was born eleven weeks prematurely on November 1, 1981, spent the first two and a half months in the hospital, and may—may—have sustained some lasting injury or handicap.

"The doctor said that he's seen babies who've come out of this all right and some that haven't. We'll have to wait and see." She speaks in a soft voice and gestures with fine-boned fingers. She has a long face, almost oval-shaped, and as she listens, more than when she speaks, she tilts it to one side. The first time we talked was in her Falls Church, Virginia, living room, which they are slowly repainting in a pleasing eggshell white. With a few pertinent details she brought me up-to-date. "I was born in 1951 in Hartford, Connecticut; my father was a business executive and my mother a housewife. My mother had had two miscarriages before me and one after me. I'm the only child. Dale and I have been married for three years." Her husband is a technical representative for a building automation company.

Carol found out she was DES-exposed in 1973 after her father read about its association with cancer in a Hartford paper. "When Daddy called I didn't think much about it, because not much was known about it." She went to a "granddaddy-type doctor," who reassured her for one solid year that she had no evidence of DES-related problems.

But when her regular doctor was away she was examined by his younger associate, who took one look at her and said, "I can see with the naked eye that you have a case of adenosis—you've got to be examined by a specialist." "That scared the hell out of me," Carol added. A Washington, D.C., specialist then told her she had moderate adenosis and performed cryosurgery three times as well as taking numerous biopsies.

Cryosurgery is a technique in which cervical tissue is frozen but not removed from the body. It is regarded today by many doctors as bad practice for DES daughters, because it can cause stenosis, or closure, of the cervix, which can also interfere with fertility. It has been criticized in at least one medical article as carrying far more risks for the DES daughter's ultimate health than the procedure itself might cure. One physician in an interview called it "meddlesome midwifery." Only a few short years ago it was recommended as, in effect, "the latest thing" for DES daughters.

Carol went frequently to doctors, who were keeping an eye out for potential cancer development. "It was a big deal when I went only once every three months." She shared her agony with her parents, with Dale, and with their friends, "but we didn't share the same experiences. They weren't DES-exposed." Later she gained a great deal of emotional strength by working as a volunteer with a consumer group, DES Action.

In 1978 Carol's mother was diagnosed as having breast cancer.

"We decided to have a baby right away, before Mom died. It became an obsession with me," Carol Simpson said. On a vacation on Cape Cod in September 1979 she stopped using birth control methods "and expected to get pregnant right away." She didn't. And didn't for a year after that.

"The doctor told me I was too emotional because of my mother. He said tests weren't needed yet, but Dale had a fertility evaluation, and came away with an acceptable sperm count, which secretly disappointed me, because I was hoping it would be him. It wasn't."

"She worried about her DES exposure but didn't really talk about it. She kept a lot of it to herself," Dale said.

On Memorial Day, 1981, Carol Simpson had her first morning sickness. Then she had a sonogram (a procedure in which sound waves are used to "picture" the baby) because of light bleeding. "I saw her heartbeat! Then later there was heavy bleeding, which the doctor said might have been due to a polyp, and he told me if I miscarried, it would look like chicken skin and to pick it out and put it in a baggie for analysis."

After celebrating with Dale, she told her mother. "Her problems seemed to go away and she said she was feeling better. She had been classically guilty [and thought] that she had caused all these problems. She *wanted* her breast cancer to be from DES. I told her it was something we had to live with, that she had wanted me, and I was here, and that if I died tomorrow I was glad I had had a good life."

On October 30, 1981, Carol experienced ruptured membranes and was rushed to Georgetown University Hospital, in Washington, D.C. "Two days after I got into the hospital I developed an infection. My white blood cell count went way up, my temperature went to about a hundred and one degrees, and I went into a natural labor." Elizabeth was born at 10:54 P.M., November 1, 1981—eleven weeks short of a full-term delivery.

Because of the premature birth the baby was whisked away for intensive care. "In the middle of the second night they told me she had had a seizure, blood had gone to the brain, the cause was unknown. She also suffered from hyaline membrane disease—which is prematurity of the lungs—and fluid between the lungs and the chest wall, which they were draining out. They were worried about her getting my infection, so they put her on antibiotics, but it seemed to have been an unnecessary precaution. The day after Thanksgiving there was more surgery—they put in a 'reservoir' under her scalp to collect the extra fluid. An improvement was seen, and they stopped tapping her." Later a permanent shunt was connected from Elizabeth's head to her abdominal cavity to keep the excess fluid drained away. She immediately began infant stimulation sessions, and Carol said her outlook is good.

Carol Simpson has worked as a medical secretary and has gone over these days with her doctors and her husband time and time again. We talked further when the baby was two months old, and Carol spoke with the same calmness and softness she had displayed in our interview months earlier in her living room. "The doctors have been fantastic, but they've been only concerned with her medical problems, especially hydrocephalus"—a medical term indicating the excessive fluid in the brain area which can cause brain and body dysfunctions, seizures, mental slowness, and poor motor coordination. As a mother, however, Carol saw things differently.

"Because of [the doctors'] concern, we had to convince them to give her more food. When she was born she weighed three pounds, two ounces, but soon she was down to two pounds, nine ounces. I had pumped"—that is, used a small machine to mechanically pump her breast milk into bottles for later use—"and she started eating two cc's at each feeding early on. Right now" (slightly more than two months after her birth) "she's at four pounds, eight and a half ounces, and climbing right up there."

Carol says she and the doctors won't know for quite some time whether their efforts have staved off any long-range problems. "But," she asked, "have I told you she's cute? She's really neat.

"The doctor said my uterus and cervix appeared to be normal, and in that sense the premature birth was not related to DES. He said most likely I delivered prematurely because of the subacute infection in the amniotic sac, which caused the water to break" (leading to the early but natural labor). "I asked him what caused the infection, and he said, 'Infections just happen.' "

Several months before Carol's baby was born the National Institutes of Health published an article in the September 1981 issue of their journal. The study was conducted at the National Institute of Environmental Health Sciences, a branch of the Department of Health and Human Services. According to the study (written by scientists Jack H. Dean, Michael Luster, and Gary A. Boorman), animals treated with DES ". . . were less able to summon biological defenses against bacteria and bacterial toxins [than nontreated animals].

"The investigators found that DES-treated animals had a lowered number of lymphoid cells in the thymus and bone marrow, key sites in the production and activity of these cells. They also saw a marked decrease in the animal's ability to ward off parasites, tumor cells, bacteria, and toxins."

In animals, as in humans, the immune system protects the body from disease: elevated temperatures and other symptoms of illness are a sign a fight is going on. Agents that assist the body in maintaining health are often developed in the thymus regions. The report says that the study was begun to investigate ways "in which environmental agents suppress the body's immune system."

In the Herbst-Bern textbook, Phyllis B. Blair, Ph.D. (professor of immunology at the University of California at Berkeley), wrote a section on the immunologic consequences of early DES exposure on rodents, which were selected and studied with a view toward implications in people.

"The brain, pituitaries, ovaries and vagina [in animals] have been identified as the main target areas of perinatally [just after birth] introduced DES, . . . and other tissues, such as the mammary gland, can be significantly affected. The immune system can now be added to this list, since it is also altered by treatment . . . Immunologic impairment can be dramatic, and it can persist through the life of the animal," Blair stated.

"The immune system undergoes a series of significant developmental changes" at a time in animals comparable to when DES is being taken by a pregnant woman. "Thus, agents administered during this sensitive period may alter the emergence and function of mature lymphocytes" (a major component of the immune system). In rodents treated with DES, Blair wrote, various cells involved in the immune system were weakened. "Another component of the immune system, natural killer cells, is also diminished; the response is lower than that of normal mice and it cannot be augmented by treatment." In other words, in these tests, even the administration of certain chemicals could not reverse the DES-related changes.

Comparing mice treated with steroid hormones and mice treated with DES, a nonsteroidal estrogen, Blair's study found that the impairment of animals treated with the steroids "is less dramatic than that found by us and others after treatment with DES." Blair listed twenty studies conducted around the world, including twelve authored or coauthored by Terje Kalland, M.D., from the University of Bergen's Institute of Anatomy, in Norway, which showed the impact of DES on the immune system of mice. Two papers were published in 1978, the rest in 1979 and 1980.

This was the conclusion to Blair's paper, which like the NIH study above, represents the cutting edge of knowledge:

> The immunologic observations on the [rodent] model system are likely to be relevant to the human, since female mice treated perinatally with DES or sex steroids exhibit reproductive tract changes similar to those of women exposed prenatally [before birth] to DES. There is thus reason for concern that the offspring of women who have received hormone therapy while pregnant or who have continued to take oral contraceptives while unknowingly pregnant may be at risk for damage not only to their reproductive systems but also to their immune system. The consequences of this damage may not become apparent for years.

Did Carol Simpson's DES exposure make her more susceptible to infections, the infections that *caused* the premature birth? At the moment no one knows. Such a conclusion could be reached only after controlled studies involving people duplicated by other scientists using animals, and controlled studies or analyses of people with documented

DES-exposure. But regarding DES, physicians and researchers all over the country continually make the same statement when asked whether DES could cause this or be associated with that: "We don't know."

In the 1980 DESAD paper mentioned earlier, showing that DES daughters in its study were at nearly twice the risk for a premature delivery as were unexposed women, there was this chilling statement: "At present one cannot determine what additional burden exposure to DES places on a pregnant woman. There remains the possibility that some as yet unrecognized selection bias or unidentified combination of confounding variables accounts for the differences. Clearly, the story is just beginning to unfold, and it may take many more years, perhaps the next decade, to obtain satisfactory answers to many of the relevant questions."

"... *confounding variables* ..."

Perhaps no truer phrase was ever written on the subject of just what DES does to people.

Shortly after Elizabeth Cady Simpson was born on November 1, 1981, Carol Simpson telephoned her mother in Hartford, who lay dying from the complications of cancer. "She went unconscious shortly after getting the news and died on December third," Carol said. "I'm glad she knew about her granddaughter."

9

MISCARRIAGES AND INFERTILITY

There is dispute in the medical community as to whether DES daughters are at a greater risk for miscarriages and infertility than nonexposed women. The differences *may* have to do with the average doses taken by mothers of women in each study, the length of time they took the drug, and a wide variety of other factors. The studies themselves focus on women whose mothers were given clearly specified amounts of DES during pregnancy. As we saw in an earlier chapter, mothers in the University of Chicago study in the 1950s were given a large amount of DES, compared to women investigated by the nationwide DESAD project. Unless a woman knows how much DES her mother took during pregnancy—and many can't find out at all, much less determine the precise dosage—she may not be able to tell which study has the most relevance to her. The differing conclusions, therefore, reflect one of the greatest problems facing DES-exposed people: not being exactly sure just what they are at risk for.

Miscarriages

A 1980 study from the University of Chicago, based on the daughters of women given the drug during the famous 1950s experiment, shows that DES daughters in that study had nearly a four times greater incidence of miscarriages and other pregnancy problems, such as stillbirth, neonatal death (death just after birth), and ectopic pregnancy (pregnancy outside the uterus) than unexposed women in the study. Only 67 percent of the DES daughters became pregnant, while 86 percent of the nonexposed women had pregnancies.

This study was published in the February 1980 issue of the *Journal of Reproductive Medicine.* Arthur L. Herbst, M.D., Marian M. Hubby, Ph.D., Richard R. Blough, M.S., and Freidoon Azizi, M.D., compared 226 DES daughters with 203 women whose mothers had not been given the drug during William Dieckmann's 1950 study. In one section, looking only at the outcome of first pregnancies for 89 DES daughters compared to 118 unexposed women, the study found that 31 percent of these DES-exposed women had either a premature nonviable baby (one that died shortly after birth), a miscarriage, or an ectopic pregnancy, compared to only 8 percent of such consequences in the unexposed group. Within those figures there were 12 miscarriages among the DES daughters and 6 among the unexposed. And 47 percent of the DES women had full-term live births, compared to 85 percent of the nonexposed women.

But in another analysis of the same figures, the authors stated that of 42 women with apparent fertility problems, 23 later became pregnant. "The reasons for the higher rate of infertility among the exposed in this study are not known, and the frequency of such factors as pelvic inflammatory disease or the husband's semen quality has not been determined. A more detailed investigation of the clinical findings and test results for these patients is needed."

Overall, 82 percent of the DES group had had at least one live offspring, compared to 93 percent of the unexposed group.

Another study, again from the Herbst group, was published in the December 15, 1981, issue of the *American Journal of Obstetrics and Gynecology.* It analyzed the outcome of a first pregnancy for 150 DES-exposed women, compared to 181 nonexposed women. Twenty-one percent of the DES women had spontaneous abortions (or miscarriages), compared to 11 percent of the unexposed group.

The mothers in the Chicago study had taken a mean dosage of 12,-031 milligrams of DES during their pregnancies. By contrast, the mean dosage of DES taken by mothers of women in the DESAD project was considerably lower, often as much as 75 percent lower than that taken by mothers in the Chicago study.

In the March 13, 1980, issue of the *New England Journal of Medicine,* the DESAD project published a paper stating that for daughters in its study, "Fertility, measured in terms of pregnancies achieved, did not differ between the women exposed to DES and the controls." Before going into some of the details of that study, it would be well to quote from one of its precisely documented tables. This one correlated the pregnancy outcome of a daughter with the amount of DES taken by her mother. As we saw in an earlier chapter, the DES daughters who had had premature births had been exposed to 3,490 milligrams of DES; DES daughters without premature birth experiences had been exposed to 2,415 milligrams. DES daughters who had had miscarriages had been exposed to 2,497.5 milligrams, while DES daughters who had never had a miscarriage had, paradoxically, been exposed to 2,520 milligrams. DES daughters who had never had a full-term live birth had been exposed to 5,260 milligrams; those who were not in that category had been exposed to 2,427.5 milligrams. Finally, women who had had any unfavorable pregnancy outcome had been exposed to 3,637.5 milligrams, while those who had not had any unfavorable outcome had been exposed to the smallest mean dosage of all, only 1,685 milligrams.

This was the same paper that spoke of "confounding variables" possibly accounting for the various pregnancy experiences of the woman surveyed.

In the 1980 DESAD paper it was found that 57 of the 220 DES-exposed women (or 25.9 percent) had had miscarriages, compared to 36 (or 16.1 percent) of the 224 unexposed women. However, because the numbers were so small, the authors stated that the risk of miscarriage for DES daughters in the study was "not statistically significant." That is a phrase used to balance the appearance that raw numbers can create against the mathematical certainty that the same percentages would appear in a much larger group. Among all women who became pregnant, 81 percent of the DES group had one full-term live birth, compared to 95 percent of the unexposed group.

The report pointed out that another factor that might have a bearing on the unsuccessful pregnancies but that had not yet been explored was the role of fathers. The authors added: "Genetic factors may never be sorted out because of the incomplete and imprecise nature of prenatal histories in the era of DES usage."

The 1981 paper from the Herbst group was the first anywhere to make a definitive statement about ectopic pregnancies (a type of pregnancy in which the egg is fertilized on or in a fallopian tube and that always ends in a miscarriage): DES-exposed daughters had a statistically significant increase in ectopic pregnancies compared to women in the control group. In that study, comparing 122 DES daughters with 141 unexposed controls, there were 12 ectopic pregnancies among the DES group, or 5.7 percent, compared to only one among the controls, or 0.3 percent. The reasons are not known.

The 1981 publication date of that finding is of value in establishing how such knowledge evolves. In his 1980 paper Herbst had pointed out that four DES daughters had had ectopic pregnancies, while none of the unexposed had had one. However, the numbers involved were not large enough for the group to state that this was statistically significant and, in effect, not coincidental. One year later, however, the ectopic pregnancy figure appeared again, this time in a large enough sample so the figure could be called, with the finest of precision, "statistically significant."

Other researchers have noted the increase in ectopic pregnancies too. In the 1980 DESAD figures there were eight ectopic pregnancies among the DES group and only three among the controls, but the numbers were not large enough to be "statistically significant."

Medical World News reported in its June 8, 1981, issue that researchers at Yale University had seen withered fallopian tubes in eleven DES daughters, and quoted a Cornell University gynecologist as wondering whether the withered or misshapen fallopian tubes might be related to the ectopic pregnancies. Ectopic pregnancies can endanger the life of the mother when they lead to a rupture of the fallopian tube. Ruptured tubal pregnancies are a leading cause of maternal death, the magazine stated. Another publication also indicated that DES daughters had a higher rate of miscarriages than did nonexposed women but that chances for a successful pregnancy increased with subsequent pregnancies. Published in the July 1981 issue of *Obstetrics and Gynecology*, the paper (whose lead author was Norma P. Veridiano, M.D., a staff physician at Brookdale Hospital Medical Center, Brooklyn, New York) followed 106 DES-exposed daughters who had a total of 159 pregnancies. There were 25 spontaneous abortions in the group, 12 premature births (one died), 60 elective abortions before the thirteenth week, 2 ectopic pregnancies, 3 women who were still pregnant at the time of the study, and 57 term births. The report indicated spontaneous abortions, or miscarriages, in DES-exposed women were more frequent than would be expected for unexposed women.

All of the patients were followed up for successive pregnancies while in the study, which concluded: "There is a trend towards a spontaneous increase in the duration of each pregnancy, an optimistic indication

that the majority of these women will eventually have a term pregnancy
. . . DES female progeny should be counseled concerning the possibility
of future impaired reproductive performance. Before they conceive
again," the study advised, they should be thoroughly examined, and
their doctors should be made aware of their DES exposure and any anatomic or structural changes.

"If pregnancy occurs before counseling and if the pregnancy attains
term status, the patient may be reassured that future reproductive performance will not be compromised as a result of her exposure to DES,"
the paper stated. In other words, according to *this* study, DES daughters as a whole have more miscarriages than nonexposed women but a
better chance at having a baby with successive attempts.

A small study in 1980 from the University of California at San Diego
also concludes that there is no significant difference in the ability of
DES daughters to get pregnant or carry to term.

The irony for DES daughters, of course, is that although their mothers took the drug to prevent miscarriages, some of the daughters have
had miscarriages and others may be at a greater risk for them.

Cynthia Hunkele regularly goes on camera to interview guests on
station WALB-TV, in Albany, Georgia, an agricultural and small business town in Georgia's southwestern red-clay region. As Woman's
Director of the station she likes to conduct her interviews on the patio
in back of the main studio, and if the Chevy-sized gnats don't get you,
her thoughtful questions will. On several occasions she has held
on-camera discussions of DES.

"It's a hard topic for me to talk about," she said after the birth of her
first child. To understand the magnitude of the DES nightmare, it
might be well to stop off in Albany, Georgia, and visit with Cynthia
Hunkele and her mother. Only when understood in the context of
something that happened in places throughout the country wherever
trucks could deliver pharmaceutical supplies, drug-company salesmen
could call at clinics, or physicians could get their free medical journals
through the mail—a town such as Albany, Georgia—will the DES story
be understood in its full power.

Albany is due south of Atlanta, and about forty-nine miles down the
road from Plains, the home of former President Jimmy Carter. Peanuts
are a major crop, nothing draws a crowd better than a softball game on
a hot afternoon, and there are cooks down there who can do more with
locally cured ham, or beans, or anything that grows in that rich soil than
you can dream of.

It was into that fragrant life that Cynthia Cannon was born on January 3, 1956. Just before her marriage, twenty-one years later, she went in for her first gynecological examination. The doctor interrupted the exam to ask her one question: Had her mother taken DES during pregnancy? A little frightened, Cynthia called her mother, Opal R. Cannon, then a teacher and now principal of the Lee County Elementary School, and was told that she had.

"Of course, I'd never had a miscarriage before when I was given it. I'd just had some bleeding during the second month with Cynthia," Mrs. Cannon said. Which is to say that DES, a drug theoretically intended for women with problems of habitual miscarriage, had been given—"and in massive doses," Mrs. Cannon remembers—to a woman who had never had a miscarriage. Bleeding during pregnancy could have indicated a host of causes, many of them unrelated to potential miscarriage.

Troubled, Cynthia went for further examination by a gynecologist, who used a colposcope, a powerful specialized microscope often used with DES daughters to determine if there are unusual cell developments in the vagina. The expensive colposcopic exam often replaces the more standard Pap smear. It was found that Cynthia had adenosis and a T-shaped uterus (instead of a uterus with the standard Y shape) as well as an improperly developed, or "incompetent," cervix.

Mrs. Cannon—and millions of other DES mothers—was given DES during the early months of pregnancy, when the uterus, vagina, and cervix are still developing within the human embryo. The shape of Cynthia's reproductive tract was apparently affected by her mother's DES medication, and the miscarriage of Cynthia's first pregnancy would be directly related to the shape of her reproductive tract.

"When I got married on July 30, 1977, I was scared to death I wouldn't be able to have children. I didn't understand it, and neither did my husband." But eleven months after their wedding, in June of 1978, Cynthia became pregnant. The pregnancy lasted for more than twenty weeks, until October 25, 1978, when the twenty-two-year-old woman started to hemorrhage in the ladies' room of the firm where she worked.

"There had been some spotting at the beginning of the pregnancy, but a sonogram showed everything was okay. About two days before the miscarriage I knew something was wrong. We called the doctor that night, but he just said, 'Well, it's probably just discharge. If it doesn't go away call me back.'" The couple's first fetus had in fact dropped down, due either to the T-shaped uterus or to the incompetent cervix, both of which are now known, in the shorthand of the medical profession, as DES stigmata. Later, in the hospital, under heavy medication, the complete miscarriage took place.

There have been a number of studies showing that DES women with these structural changes tend to have a higher rate of miscarriages than women without the changes. Researchers point out that other aspects of being a DES daughter, either hormonal or endocrinological, could also be involved.

Cynthia sighed as she talked: "After the miscarriage I felt restless. I felt incompetent as a woman. I [felt I had] let everyone down, including myself. I couldn't do what I was put here on earth to do. A woman can do much more of course, but we can also have babies, and I couldn't."

Several women who admire Cynthia Hunkele's personal and professional capabilities recall that her weight went up following the miscarriage and that she seemed constantly depressed and morose. She does not have these recollections but acknowledges it might have appeared that way to others.

In February of 1979 she started her position as Woman's Director at the Albany TV station. In late 1980 she became pregnant for the second time. But it was not without a great deal of thought and worry. "I had been putting it off because I was scared I might have to spend nine months in bed. I had mixed emotions, but I was willing to do what I had to do. This time I went to the doctor every two weeks for an exam, and during the last eight weeks I went on a weekly basis. I kept working part-time until July 31—two and a half weeks before the baby was born. I took it easy."

She also got some sophisticated medical treatment. Her doctor put in a cervical stitch to correct and strengthen her cervix, whose failure to maintain its rigidity had apparently contributed to her earlier miscarriage. The stitch, which has now become common practice for women with unusually shaped cervixes, was put in at the third month of pregnancy (the miscarriage had occurred near the end of the fourth month).

Joseph Martin Hunkele, Jr., was born on August 20, 1981, after a Caesarean section. He weighed seven pounds, four and one-half ounces. His mother pronounces him "extremely healthy."

The simple cervical stitch, an inexpensive and possible lifesaver, is still in place. "If I ever have any more kids I'll be ready," she said.

She has gotten answers to questions she has asked physicians but has also been told there is a great deal that isn't known. "I do resent like hell that they did this, made this drug. My mother was a guinea pig, and so was I." She is not the only DES daughter in the tiny town of Albany, Georgia. "A lot of my friends are DES-exposed too. Some of them are starting to have trouble."

Susan Lawler had three miscarriages before the birth of her son in 1980. Susan and her husband, Francis X. Lawler, were born in Philadelphia in 1956 and now live in a nearby suburb. Frannie Lawler's story will be told in the chapter on DES sons.

"My mother had had two children, then a miscarriage, when she became pregnant with me. But I didn't find out that she'd taken DES until 1975, after I had my first miscarriages," Susan said.

When she was seventeen Susan was told by a doctor that she had polyps on her cervix, which was rare for a woman so young. The polyps were removed. Then a cervical band was discovered, and removed, and reconstructive surgery was done on the cervix. These conditions have all been associated in women with DES use during pregnancy by their mothers. Susan has also had five D and C's (dilatation and curettage), a medical procedure that removes tissue from the lining of the cervical canal and from the endometrial cavity.

"In 1975 I had a miscarriage, and then six months later, in 1976, I had another miscarriage. I called my mother's doctor, and he told me he had given my mother DES. She started taking it in the third month, and took it until the end of pregnancy, ten milligrams a day. My mother felt real guilty. She said, 'I only took it because they said without it I'd have another miscarriage,' " Susan remembered.

There was a third pregnancy and a third miscarriage in 1978, and then a fourth, and successful, pregnancy in 1980. "During my pregnancy there was a lot of fear. Every time I caught a cold everyone panicked. In my seventh month there was a false labor, and then Keith was born, on September 19, 1980. My exposure is minimal compared to others', but it's been a struggle."

Laura Minor is twenty-six years old, a physician's assistant in Los Angeles. She and her husband, Craig, a graduate student of urban planning, live in an apartment in the Gardena section of the city.

Laura started taking birth control pills when she was fifteen to control her excessive menstrual cramps each month, and used the pill, on and off, until she was twenty. Since age eighteen she has suffered from bladder problems, and a recent biopsy found squamous metaplasia in her bladder. Metaplasia is a condition in which mature cells change into abnormal shapes, which could be an indication of potential problems. Her mother took DES during her pregnancy with Laura, who was born in 1956.

In late January 1982 she miscarried her first pregnancy. "The doctor said the miscarriage was caused by a blighted ovum, that there was something wrong with the fetus itself," she said.

She has had a number of other medical problems throughout her life, particularly endometriosis (aberrant tissue in the pelvic cavity), which apparently caused blood-filled cysts in her uterus and ovaries. She recently had surgery to remove the endometriosis, and although the operation was thought to be successful, the condition has since returned. Medicine to help control the problem cost her $100 to $160 a month for six months. Insurance covers part of the cost but not all of it.

For years she has had considerable pain. Once, in 1968, as a twelve-year-old and an eighth-grade student, she lay in bed for three days, screaming. "I had terrible pains, I couldn't walk, I wanted to die." As an adult she has had symptoms similar to chronic vaginitis (an inflammation of the vagina). She *hurt.* "There was a lot of pain during intercourse—it wasn't pleasant for me or Craig. There was pain whenever I'd use tampons, tremendous pain. I went to seven or eight gynecologists, and they basically said I'd grow out of it. Not one asked about DES exposure. There was pain a good deal of the time. I'd lie awake at night and cry. My mother worked for a drug company; she said a lot of her friends were taking DES [at that time]."

When we first spoke, at her home, Laura had not yet tried to get pregnant. She had said then: "The worst thing is not knowing. Will I be able to get pregnant? Will I be able to carry to term? Will there be a recurrence of these pains, or other problems, when I go through menopause? Who knows?" After her miscarriage she wrote me a note about it. "I started spotting last Thursday and did so on and off until Monday. I saw my OB, who felt a large mass on my left side. They did an ultrasound. The baby died two weeks ago, and I have another cyst, blood-filled like the others. It was the size of a cantaloupe. I miscarried Tuesday after two and a half months. Was it DES? Who knows?"

Infertility

The 1980 University of Chicago study also developed disturbing statistics indicating that DES-exposed daughters in its investigation had a harder time getting pregnant than the nonexposed women and that there were more among them who were unable to get pregnant *at all*, than among the nonexposed women. As we will see, these conclusions are not shared by other studies, where the women involved were generally exposed to smaller amounts of DES during pregnancy.

In its 1980 paper the Herbst group examined the conception experience of 226 DES daughters and 203 unexposed controls. One section looked at the "proportion of unprotected women who have been pregnant," meaning both married and single women who had not used birth control devices and had gotten pregnant. Within that group only 67 percent of the DES daughters had gotten pregnant, as against 86 percent of the non-DES women.

The next section dealt with the "proportion of unprotected married women who have been pregnant" and found that 73 percent of the DES group had been pregnant, compared to 90 percent of the non-DES group.

Finally, a section looked at the women who had "tried unsuccessfully for a pregnancy for one year or more" and found that 42 DES-exposed women (19 percent of the total) had been unsuccessful in getting pregnant over the course of at least one year, compared to 21 unexposed women (10 percent of the total). Within the last grouping, however, was this figure: 19 DES-exposed women had never been pregnant at all, compared to only 4 women in the unexposed group.

The report stated: "The reasons for the higher rate of infertility among the exposed are not known, and the frequency of such factors as pelvic inflammatory disease [which can interfere with conception] or the husband's semen quality has not been determined." The 1981 Chicago study reached similar conclusions on the subject of fertility.

In general, researchers point out that conception is a delicate matter of an egg being released on time in the ovary, maturing in a fallopian tube, being fertilized by sperm in the upper part of the fallopian tube and then traveling (usually over a week's time) to the uterus, where the newly formed blastocyst attaches itself to the wall of the uterus, eventually forming the early stages of the placenta, in which the embryo will mature.

For all this to be happening, the body must release such substances as follicle-stimulating hormone (FSH) and luteinizing hormone (LH). These two hormones are secreted by the pituitary gland and act together to make sure the egg is released to a fallopian tube. Estrogen and progesterone are also needed to ensure the health of the ovum before fertilization takes place; after fertilization takes place, a new set of variables comes into play. At all times the reproductive areas must be moist and able to accept the fertilization process: the egg must live and move; so must the sperm. Many parts of the body are involved in delicate balances: the ovaries, fallopian tubes, uterus, the glands, the brain (which influences the release of hormones), and so on. Possibly, in the DES women experiencing an inability to get pregnant, these balances may have been upset.

Not all researchers have reached the conclusion drawn by Herbst and the Chicago group. For example, the 1980 DESAD study found that "fertility, measured in terms of pregnancies achieved, did not differ between the women exposed to DES and the controls." Comparing the fertility of 618 women exposed to DES with the fertility of 618 women who had not been exposed to it, the DESAD study found that 53.2 percent of the DES women had not been pregnant, compared to 49.8 percent of the unexposed women, and that 46.8 percent of the DES women had gotten pregnant, compared to 50.2 percent of the unexposed women. Larry Cousins, M.D., at the University of California, San Diego, also published a paper in 1980, showing that in his small study fertility did not differ between DES-exposed and unexposed women, although he too saw an increase in premature deliveries.

The differences between the studies reflect, in large part, researchers say, the differing populations being studied and, to some extent, different research methods of analysis.

It is important to focus on the statistics of the various DES studies in order to understand the magnitude of the nightmare the drug has created. But even a successful pregnancy cannot take away all of the pain associated with unsuccessfully trying for years to get pregnant, nor can the birth of a healthy baby blot out all the unhappiness of a previous miscarriage. Therefore it is equally important to focus on the people involved, among whom notably are the DES daughters who so far have been unable to have children.

"You go all through high school and college avoiding pregnancy, and then when you decide you're ready, you pick the month and season and expect it to happen just because you've now decided," Debbie Wingard said.

The soft breezes were blowing off the Pacific as we sat outside the cafeteria at the University of California at San Diego's La Jolla campus. Debbie Wingard, an epidemiologist with a Ph.D. and a faculty position in the school's Department of Community and Family Medicine, was awaiting her first baby. She would not be the baby's biological mother, however, though she would be its emotional and adoptive mother; she and her husband, an attorney, were planning to adopt the baby of a young unmarried woman whose parents had asked her to leave their house and whom Debbie and her husband had taken in. The young woman had not wanted an abortion but also had not wanted to keep the baby, so an affectionate arrangement had been worked out: the expectant mother would live with them until the baby was born and then legally release to Debbie and here husband all rights to the child.

Debbie still had two eventualities to worry about: a safe delivery and the possibility that the young woman might have a change of heart.

The twists and turns that Debbie Wingard and her husband, Pierre Vaughn, endured are a familiar story in the DES community: making do as best you can; trying to improve on a situation you didn't ask for and shouldn't have had to expect; having guts; having courage; having love.

"I was a student at U.C. Berkeley in 1975 when I learned during a routine exam about possible DES exposure, which my mother confirmed through records. I've got adenosis [atypical cells seen during a colposcopy exam], a Type 2 cervix, fibrous bands around my cervix, and a slightly T-shaped uterus. My fallopian tubes are normal. Even as a professional using statistics I knew that the cancer risk was low, but it was still an upsetting thing. Every time I went in for an exam—twice a year—I expected it to be worse than it was. I was afraid of cancer."

In theory, Debbie should have been able to get pregnant, but somehow it never happened.

"We decided to have kids after I finished graduate school, and I assumed once we started trying, it would be only a few months. My period was regular and there didn't seem to be any problem, but I wasn't getting pregnant. In 1978 I went to a specialist and in the course of the exam told him I was a DES daughter. He said that he'd started to hear that some DES daughters were having problems getting pregnant. This was the first time I had heard of fertility problems being related to DES, and then I started getting mad. I realized how little was known about the subject."

At the same time her husband went to a urologist, and he discovered that he had a low sperm count. "In fact, Pierre, who is diabetic, wonders if he's DES-exposed too, but he's never been able to find out directly." Low sperm counts can occur in DES sons, although they can also occur in diabetic men who are not DES-exposed.

Debbie brushes her shoulder-length hair back from her face. "I started temperature-monitoring of my cycle [a technique used in part to find the optimal moment for getting pregnant], and discovered I had a beautiful, classic temperature cycle. We thought the problem might be the low sperm count, so we tried artificial insemination from anonymous donors. We tried cervical insemination, vaginal insemination, and uterine insemination, but nothing worked." These procedures, which occasionally produced "cramping so severe I thought I was going to die," are part of the new arsenal in fertility medicine to assist in the union of a sperm and an egg. They attempt to bypass whatever structural or biological problems are interfering with conception.

"One doctor," Debbie said, "*thought* I had an unusually small amount of cervical mucus, which might keep the sperm from being properly transported. He wanted to use estrogens to increase the mucus, and here I started empathizing with my mother: I wanted a baby so badly, and she had too; she just didn't have the knowledge that I had . . . I took some estrogen, Premarin [a natural product made from the substances found in pregnant mare's urine] before ovulation, because that way, if I got pregnant, it wouldn't be around to harm the baby. That didn't work either."

She stayed on the treadmill of medical visits. One doctor told her she had a high level of prolactin, one of the body's hormones, which *might* mean she had a tumor or tumors on her pituitary gland, which could be suppressing the release of hormones needed for conception. She was also told she had a "disorganized" endometrium that contained cells in all stages of development. One doctor treated her with Clomid, a fertility drug that raised the risk of a multiple birth. Then Debbie was told that Clomid decreased estrogens, which she needed for pregnancy, so she added estrogens to her medical menu.

She did not get pregnant.

"I received very good, very concerned, medical care. The physician was extra sensitive to me because his wife is a DES daughter. But nothing worked."

Her physician suggested they think about adoption while they went through further fertility tests. "How we got children didn't concern me very much," said Pierre Vaughn. "The method didn't matter—whether it was artificial insemination or adoption, whatever. We like children. We wanted children. It makes your family complete."

"This was 1979," Debbie went on, "and an adoption agency told us it would take at least five years. But we were also told it might be difficult because Pierre is blind, a result of his diabetes. He lost his sight in 1976, a year after our marriage." Pierre added, "You spend some time cursing the stars, but that doesn't get you anywhere. You get on with your life."

They tried a mass mailing, hoping to find a baby nobody wanted, but that had no results. Then they began working with a lawyer married to an adoption counselor in another California city. The only definite criteria Debbie and Pierre had were that they wanted a healthy baby and they wanted a Caucasian baby. "We preferred a Caucasian baby because we have enough problems with other aspects of our life," she said.

The attorney brought them together with the young woman who was now living with them. She was eighteen years old.

"We flew her down to San Diego. We all got along very well. The girl's parents had asked her to leave the house, and she didn't want to live by herself. We agreed to have her live with us and to pay her living expenses. Even after the baby's born she's got six months to change her mind about giving the baby up. She's due any day now."

That was in July 1981. On August 21 baby Brendan was born, weighing eight pounds and five ounces. The child was delivered after a marathon forty-hour labor, with Debbie Wingard serving as the girl's labor coach for the natural childbirth. Shortly after the birth the young woman became reconciled with her parents, and after a tearful goodbye to the Wingards she rejoined her family, while Brendan began life with his new family.

"I personally feel DES has a lot to do with my fertility problems. I have a low mucus, he has a low sperm count. When you have these problems you don't mind each step. The problems themselves don't frighten me. But there's a point where one medical problem comes along after another, and it gets to be very frustrating. You get the feeling, I'm not going to solve this one, then you spend a couple of hours crying and you feel better," Debbie said.

"All the tests indicate that I do not ovulate," Pamela Mills Fink said. Born on February 1, 1948, in Astoria, Oregon, she now lives with her husband, a construction company executive, in a spanking new townhouse in West Covina, California. She is an accomplished weaver whose complex textiles adorn the whitewashed walls of her home.

"I have one ovary that is in a 'resting' condition, which means it isn't working, and the other one is trying to work but hasn't. The doctors feel it is a hormone problem, that something is interfering with the signals being sent from the brain. Pretty soon I'm going to start in a program trying to correct this."

She wasn't worried when she found out about her exposure in 1975, although she began to wonder whether this drug might somehow be linked to the "excessive and prolonged bleeding" that began shortly after she started menstruating at age twelve and was once so bad it required hospitalization and three pints of blood. In 1976, however, she learned that she had extensive adenosis, a slight cervical cockscomb, and a patch of glandular cells on the cervix. In 1978 and 1981 she had surgery for endometrial cysts in the pelvic cavity.

"My mother had no problems getting pregnant, but I do, and I'm a DES daughter. *We've been trying to get pregnant for four and a half years.* DES daughters do have a higher rate of anovulation [the absence of ovulation]. I'd like to know why." She paused. "I've had a couple of years of being really scared and angry about it. I felt there was something going on with my body and no one had answers to it. But it was my body, damn it, and I wanted to know!

"I got involved with DES Action in Portland, Oregon, and also down here, and that has helped vent my anger some. But I've come in touch with my own mortality because of this; I've lain awake at night, worrying, and then been angry in the daytime because nothing is being done. My husband, while sympathetic, is not threatened by my DES exposure, but the pain from endometriosis affects my sex life. I know there's never been any connection made between DES and endometriosis, but will there be someday? Sometimes I wish I didn't know so much about the subject."

The program she is about to enter will attempt to stimulate her brain into releasing the luteinizing hormone, which in effect ripens the egg and makes it receptive for fertilization.

Pam Fink has lived with her body's problems for six years now, watching her friends get pregnant, watching herself unable to have a child, watching herself become a part of the American medical process.

As we sat at the oak table in her dining area she made a statement that has come to sum up for me what so many DES-exposed women— and men—feel. We were talking about the efforts of various consumer groups to pass legislation that would establish DES screening clinics and educational programs for people just learning about their exposure, programs conducted in a community setting that would offer advice and information. Her voice was steady but trembled at its edges, and tears gathered in her eyes. "I can accept having exams for the rest of my life, taking off my clothes in front of yet another strange doctor (though this gets harder each time), but why is there such resistance to recognizing the need for DES legislation and clinics, and medical and emotional help for the millions of us unwitting victims of medical research? Why?"

Michael Jardina has dreams and they trouble him. "Since we've known about Marie's DES involvement, I've had this dream. In my dream my wife dies. This is hard for me to talk about. I love her dearly . . ."

The Jardinas live in Reistertown, Maryland, an outlying suburb of Baltimore. She's a lover of Shakespeare and, at age twenty-seven, a research and development lab technician. Michael is the business manager for a local car dealership.

"This has brought us closer together, I can tell you that. We know we can survive by ourselves."

Marie has adenosis, cervical erosion, uterine hyperplasia (an overgrowth of tissue inside the womb), a T-shaped uterus, one fallopian tube that is very small and variegated (unusually marked), and a small vagina that produces occasional pain during intercourse. Marie and Michael have tried for three years to get pregnant. "The doctors say possibly the T-shaped uterus is keeping implantation from taking place. But they don't really know. We're still trying. I don't like being infertile, but it beats the hell out of cancer."

Marie's mother took twenty-two pills each day for the first four months of her pregnancy with Marie. The pills were DES, vitamins, progesterone, and thyroid pills. Marie was born on Mary 11, 1954, in Windber, Pennsylvania, which is eighty miles southeast of Pittsburgh. She had her first period at the age of twelve, and when she was thirteen and in the seventh grade she was put on the birth control pill to control menstrual irregularities.

As a young married woman of twenty she experienced a miscarriage, despite the fact that she was again on birth control pills, this time to prevent pregnancy. She experienced extreme agony and suffering, and a cold shoulder from a woman doctor who reprimanded her for calling at home after Marie had found skinlike remains in her bed following the miscarriage. Not until two more doctors had examined her following this experience did she learn of the condition of her uterus, cervix, and fallopian tube.

Since that time, despite years of trying, the Jardinas have not been able to achieve a pregnancy.

"It's certainly a blow to your ego," Marie explained, "not being able to have kids. It's difficult for my husband, sometimes he goes on a guilt trip, saying it's *his* fault—"

"Maybe *I'm* DES exposed," Michael adds. "I've had my sperm count checked, and it's OK, but who knows?"

"I do feel sometimes I'm letting him down. I could understand if he left to find someone who could have children. It would devastate me if he did, but I don't want him to be bitter in forty or fifty years that he never had children. He says children have never mattered that much, but I wonder . . ."

"At the beginning of the marriage I didn't want children, then I did, and then I realized that apparently we couldn't have them. But her health is the most important thing to me. She's had this lingering, low-grade temperature now for months."

"I try to vent my anger," Marie says. "I'm working with two young girls who've just found out they're exposed. But I do get frustrated. My friend just had her third baby in four years. I think I've handled it well. I know I'm okay on the surface, at least, but not inside when I see some-one walk by who's pregnant. We've looked into adoption, but I don't know if it's worth it for us. I don't tell people about my DES exposure, because I don't want their pity, I don't want to be treated like a freak."

Right now it is the lingering illness of unknown origins that saps much of her strength and spirit. "There are two-centimeter nodes under my left arm, and a small cluster under my right, and a small group in my groin area. There's a rash on my legs and knees all the time and a rash that comes and goes on my upper arms and elbows," she said. No one so far has provided a medical explanation for her constant low-grade fever or the rashes. "I check out as normal on the fanciest tests they've got."

I asked her about the costs of her medical examinations. "The total's been over ten thousand dollars, though insurance picks up eighty percent of that. It's a lot of money, but it would be worth it if it brought good health. No amount of money can compensate for the loss of good health," she said.

Her health has been undermined in another way too. "A doctor recently said that after all my tests I should see a psychiatrist, that this was all my fault, all in my head." She did consult a psychologist, who concluded that "there is no evidence to support a theory of hypochondria or psychosomatic illness. The patient is an intelligent and fairly well-adjusted individual." She paused. "I think that's typical of some people, some doctors, that when they can't find a cure for you they put the blame on you rather than themselves.

"The one good sign," Marie Jardina said, "is that one doctor said he has seen worse cases than me who have still had children."

10
DES SONS

In years past David McWaters has felt pain when he urinated or during sexual intercourse. He has a history of urethral problems (problems with the passage through which urine is discharged from the bladder) and infections of the prostate gland, which surrounds the urethra and bladder in men. Such problems have been associated with men exposed *in utero* to DES. He is one of them.

But David McWaters, a graduate student of pharmacy at the University of California at San Francisco, also has problems that have not yet been associated with DES exposure. "Half of the time during sexual intercourse my testicles will rise up and bang against the pelvic bone," he says. "It's painful and bothersome. When I was younger the problem was worse. My testicles would sit up near my abdomen, about four inches too high. When I'd cross my legs they'd rise up. I'd push them back down and hear a kind of *pop, pop* sound. When the testicles rise up above the pelvic bone they are easily hurt. I've bashed myself a couple of good ones."

No one has been able to explain what has caused this. As he talks about these matters he sighs. McWaters is a symbolic brother of the millions of DES daughters who have some unexplained malady for which no answer has been given.

The impact on sons of women who took DES is turning out to be the next major chapter in the DES saga. Just as the early 1970s were a period of concern about a potential vaginal cancer epidemic in young women, and the late 1970s were a time of concern about fertility prob-

lems in those same daughters, the 1980s are now bringing public attention to the problems of DES sons. The first federal report on DES sons
is expected to be released in late 1983, nearly five years after the first
federal report on DES daughters.

In March of 1983 the *Journal of the American Medical Association*
(JAMA) published a case report of two DES sons who had developed
testicular cancer. That marked the first time in any medical publication
that testicular cancer had been linked to DES sons. Although only two
cases were listed, the significance is that all articles in JAMA must pass
a rigorous peer review process, and the article's publication shows how
concerned physicians have become about the problem.

One reason for delayed information regarding men is that DES sons
are hard to find. Most young women visit a gynecologist as a matter of
course by the time they reach their teens or early twenties, either for a
routine examination or a premarital exam. But most men never go to a
urologist or an internist unless there is a specific problem, and the
problem may not involve checking their testicles, penis, or reproductive
tract. Moreover, men around the world grow up with the macho image
of suffering pain in silence, and do not always pay prompt attention to
symptoms that may be clues to larger problems. In addition, volunteers
in both major consumer groups report that DES mothers seem to have
a harder time talking about DES with their sons than with their daughters, and a number of DES mothers have said they read the early reports
involving women and silently thought, Thank God my child's a son!

Still another reason is that although physicians have never had trouble enlisting women for DES studies, recruiting men seems to be a different story. Many women had registered at DES clinics across the
country or had been told of their exposure by their mothers and were
used to being examined by doctors. But, according to Leonard T. Kur-
land, M.D., chairman and professor of epidemiology and statistics at
the Mayo Clinic, in order to get 300 men to participate in the federal
government's first major study of DES sons, researchers at Mayo had to
pay each man $35.

Finally, if doctors examining young men are not aware of the full
spectrum of potential problems (as a number of them I interviewed
have not been), or if the son himself is not aware he has been exposed or
refuses to talk about it, then potential problems may go unrecognized.

The DES textbook coauthored by Arthur Herbst and Howard A.
Bern contains a chapter on DES sons. Written by William B. Gill,

M.D., Ph.D., and three other researchers, the chapter summarizes the few studies done on DES sons up through 1981. Gill includes data on structural abnormalities found in the genital tracts of DES sons compared to unexposed sons, as described in Dieckmann's study at the University of Chicago and in studies at the University of Southern California, Stanford University, and Beth Israel Hospital in New York.

Gill points out that the Chicago study (published in 1979) was the largest, comparing 308 DES sons with 307 controls. It found that 8.4 percent of the DES sons had hypoplasia (incomplete development) of the testicles, compared to only 2 percent of the unexposed; that 17 DES sons had cryptorchidism (undescended testicles), compared to only one of the unexposed; and that 9 DES sons had capsular induration (a hardened or thickened area) on the testicles, compared to only 3 of the unexposed men. More than 20 percent of the DES sons had epididymal cysts (benign growths in a passageway around the testicle), compared to only 4.9 percent of the unexposed; and 4 DES sons had microphallus (small penis), compared to none of the controls.

Thirty-one percent of the DES sons had at least one of these structural abnormalities, compared to 7.8 percent of the controls. As the authors of the study state: "Whether the structural abnormalities will have effects on function has not been determined."

Gill's chapter goes on to show that there were some variations in the incidence of these abnormalities in DES sons analyzed in the other studies, and also some abnormalities that didn't appear in the Chicago group. For example, 29 percent of the DES sons in the Beth Israel study had varicoceles (varicose veins inside the testicles that can block the flow of semen and interfere with fertility). Two of 11 DES sons in the USC study had this condition; in the Stanford study, 2 DES sons had varicoceles, but so did 4 of the unexposed men. This condition can be surgically treated.

Brian Henderson, M.D., who led the USC study, found other changes in the genitalia of DES sons: 4 of 11 boys studied had meatal stenosis (an unusually narrow opening at the tip of the penis). Nearly 13 percent of the DES boys in the USC study complained of problems passing urine, compared to only 1.8 percent of the unexposed. One of the DES males in the USC study had hypospadia (in which the opening of the penis is underneath or to the side of its normal position).

Gill's textbook paper also compared semen produced by DES sons with that of unexposed men from the Chicago study. The only significant statistical difference between the semen analyses for DES sons and unexposed men was in the category of sperm motility (the ability of sperm to move spontaneously). DES sons did somewhat more poorly than the nonexposed men in this category, which can, in theory, affect fertility. The authors pointed out that some "qualitative differences between the groups did appear, in that higher proportions of the DES-exposed males had some lower semen quality features." In fact, two men in the DES group were azoospermic, meaning there was a complete lack of sperm in the semen. Regarding fertility, Gill's team concluded:

> It is too early to assess the fertility potential of the DES-exposed males, since only one-third to one-half of this population is old enough to allow evaluation of their reproductive performance . . . There are more individuals among the DES-exposed men [in the Chicago group] who have tried for more than one year to achieve pregnancy [than among the nonexposed]. A final judgment on the fertility of DES-exposed males can only be made after a majority of this population has passed several years of trying to reproduce. The association between DES exposure *in utero* and certain structural abnormalities of the male genital tract as well as certain trends towards slightly different (though not statistically significant) semen properties, suggests the advisability of careful examination of the reproductive system of individuals who were exposed to DES *in utero.*

The Stanford University study reached a different conclusion, based on its analysis of twenty-four exposed and unexposed subjects: "We . . . find no differences in psychosexual history, genital abnormalities, or semen analysis between the two groups." And a 1977 study from the University of Chicago found no statistical differences for DES sons compared to controls in such matters as age at the start of puberty, body height and weight, and other matters.

However, because other studies have noted differences in men exposed during pregnancy to DES, there has been interest in learning how DES might have affected the developing male embryo. A number of scholars feel that DES may interfere with the normal development and release of hormones and enzymes affecting male development, slowing down the masculinizing of the embryo. Although the sex of the embryo is determined at the moment of fertilization, the development of sexual characteristics does not begin until about the seventh week of life.

The cells that will eventually develop into the female reproductive tract in women spring from the müllerian ducts. The important cells for the reproductive organs in males spring from the wolffian ducts, and the müllerian (or female) ducts must be chemically told to "regress," or disappear. This is affected by the Anti-Müllerian Hormone (AMH), which comes into play at about the seventh week and is partially responsible for the developing sexual differentiation of the embryo.

It is possible that the introduction of DES suppresses or slows down the release or effectiveness of the Anti-Müllerian Hormone and so compromises the full development of the male sex organs. The cells that develop into the penis in men develop into the clitoris in women, and the cells that form the labia in women form the scrotum in men. The chemical interference produced by DES might account for such abnormalities as small penises, undescended testicles, hypospadia, varicoceles, epididymal cysts, and lowered sperm production.

Problems with male offspring could well have been anticipated by researchers in the earliest days of DES usage. In the late 1930s and early 1940s researchers Greene, Burrill, and Ivy were publishing their conclusions about the impact of estrogens on the sexual development of rats. Their well-received findings showed that in females DES crossed the placenta and affected the development of portions of the vagina; in males the epididymis, the mass of small, twisted tubes next to the testicle, was smaller than normal in rats born to DES-exposed mothers. There also was an impact on other organs of the sexual and reproductive system in rats. No study at the time, however, followed such test animals through animal life to check on their reproductive capabilities.

The DES for the Greene, Burrill, and Ivy study was provided by E. R. Squibb & Sons, which later marketed DES for use during pregnancy. Eli Lilly & Company also marketed DES. When I asked two senior company officials at Lilly headquarters in Indianapolis, Indiana, what the corporate response to such early studies had been, they stated that those studies were regarded as interesting data only and not something that should inhibit the marketing of the drug.

Dave McWaters was born in southern California on September 5, 1953, by which time several studies had already shown that DES was ineffective in preventing miscarriages. He first experienced problems with his testicles, which were fully descended at birth, in the seventh grade and asked his family pediatrician about it. "He said there was nothing he could do about it."

Dave found out about his DES exposure during a casual conversation with his mother when he was about twenty-four years old. Because of the association between DES and cancer in daughters exposed *in utero*, and the increasing incidence of testicular cancer (although there has not been an association drawn between it and DES-exposed sons) Dave, who is now married, is especially careful of his health. "I've learned the signs of testicular cancer. I do a self-exam." Those signs, which include hardening of a testicle or unusual growths, have not shown up. "I can't separate fear from paranoia," he says. "I wonder what problems I'll have later in life. I'm fertile now. Should we try to have children? Will I be more susceptible to prostate cancer as time goes on? It's amazing the myriad problems it's caused."

As a pharmacy student Dave now finds that his DES exposure has affected his attitude toward the drug industry. "The drug companies are primarily interested in making a profit. That can lead to a lot of irresponsibility. I haven't been thinking about this subject for very long. Certainly there is a core of emotionalism I haven't plumbed yet. But look, while we're sitting here [in San Francisco], the helicopters are out spraying Malathion all over the peninsula, trying to kill the medflies. Don't you think the epidemiologists will be all over the place in a few years looking for signs of what Malathion did to people there? What are we doing to our bodies?"

A man in New York City, a ranking executive in Manhattan, is currently plumbing the emotional depths David McWaters mentioned. He and his wife tried repeatedly throughout 1981 to get pregnant. "She is also DES-exposed, and after she went in for her fertility tests, which were negative, I thought I should go in for mine."

As a young man, athletic and sexually active, he had noticed large veins on his left testicle. "I was concerned about it. I asked a friend, a medical student, to examine me. He said there was nothing wrong. I think I had some fears, some psychological fears, that there might be a problem."

Last year, at thirty-three years of age, he went to a Manhattan fertility clinic. He recounts the episode with a kind of locker-room humor that it has taken him some time to apply to the subject.

"The doctor said he needed to take a sperm count, so I masturbated into a vial. I have a fertile imagination, if nothing else. Then I took it to the nurse, a large, military-type woman, who handled the vial as if it was so much saliva. 'How did you obtain this?' she asked. 'By hand,' I told her. She didn't say another word."

Two days later the doctor phoned him with the news. "He said I had a low sperm count, about four million [per milliliter]. Then I learned that the high end of the fertility scale is about eighty million, the low end about twenty million, although the doctor told me that pregnancies have resulted with a sperm count of only one million. But as things stood then, the odds were a hundred to one against a pregnancy."

The analysis confirmed a fear he had harbored much of the time. "My wife's postcoital analysis had consistently showed almost zero sperm. There's a basic masculine, macho, ego thing here. I felt deflated." But not defeated. His physician suspected that his low sperm count was due to a varicocele. Some of the sperm traveling through that constricted area become overheated and die, thus lowering the total sperm count. An operation was necessary. The procedure, expected to take less than an hour, took more than two because the varicocele "was one of the largest he had ever seen."

The night I called, he had just learned to give himself injections of human chorionic gonadotropin (HCG), which he must take twice weekly for ten weeks. "They said they don't know how it works exactly, but there's been a better success rate when these hormones are used."

As a sign of how much consciousness nonmedical people in this country have developed in recent years, this man made sure the hormones he was taking were natural hormones and not synthetic ones, like DES. "I said since DES might have done this to me, I didn't want to start the process all over again." In theory, the chances of a successful fertilization may go up as high as 40 percent, he said.

"I don't know how I feel about this. I was very upset at the start. There has been no strain on my relations with my wife, but there have been some unpleasant moments. I would react over-emotionally, I'd fly off the handle, get pissed off and yell at her. I got furious at her when she called me at work, reminding me to make an appointment with the doctor, because I'd already done it."

Other relationships may also become strained. When I asked this man about his feelings toward his mother and her role in his current medical problems, his statement echoed the feelings a few other men had expressed: he simply didn't want his mother to know about the problems, period. "I am determined my mother won't find out about this. I don't want that intrusive mothering. It would only be an opportunity for her to ask impertinent questions." I did not find any women who refused to tell their mothers about their DES-related problems, although some of them said they had anger, frustration, and difficulty in doing so.

As this is written, the man and his wife are waiting the required six months to see if his sperm count has increased and whether they can have a child. If not, they must consider a new course of action: Do they want to adopt?

"If we try to get pregnant for two years, say, that'll make us both thirty-five when we might start thinking about adoption. Maybe that'll be too old for us. We just don't know. Right now we're taking it one step at a time."

Roger Thomsen of Sacramento was born on June 22, 1949. He was exposed to DES *in utero,* and Agent Orange in Vietnam. "I have a lot of social issues to deal with, and they're all government-related," he said.

His mother, Phyllis Thomsen, had never been pregnant before. "The doctor was afraid I'd miscarry, I was having some cramping," she said.

The DES given to Phyllis Thomsen as preventive therapy for possible miscarriage is another proof that DES was nationally used in this country for everything involving pregnancy except the runny nose, and is a perfect rejoinder to DES apologists who say it was used only in late pregnancy.

Although he has not experienced any DES-related problems to date, "It's been on my mind the last couple of weeks," Roger told me. "I've been reading more about sons. I'm going to get a fertility test *soon.* I wouldn't want the chance of having a baby taken away from me."

The rate for testicular cancer in general is higher now than it has ever been, somewhere between 7 or 8 cases for each 100,000 men between the ages of twenty and thirty-four. The rate has tripled in the last ten years. Although no conclusive correlation has been found between DES exposure *in utero* and the development years later of testicular cancer, the increased number of cases has led researchers to question the association.

In the March 11, 1983 edition of the *Journal of the American Medical Association,* four physicians from Tufts-New England Medical Center in Boston described for the first time in the medical literature cases of testicular cancer found in two DES sons. One DES son was 28, the other was 27. The 28-year-old's mother had taken DES throughout her pregnancy, in amounts up to 105 milligrams each day, a fairly standard regime. The 27-year-old son had five siblings, all exposed to DES—one sister had vaginal cancer, another had adenosis, and a brother had a very low sperm count. The authors said their finding did not "prove" that DES exposure causes testicular cancer in men. "However, [they] should alert the medical community to the possibility of such an association," they stated.

The dramatic case histories of these two men were antcipated by earlier studies.

One questionnaire sought information from the patient on such things as marriage history, cigarette smoking, childhood illnesses, such as mumps and chicken pox, and surgical history, such as appendectomies, tonsillectomies, and hernia repairs. But the report stated that there were no greater risks deduced from any one of these factors for men who later developed testicular cancer.

Another questionnaire asked the mothers about their own health during the pregnancy with the son who later developed testis cancer. They were asked about cramping, bleeding, high blood pressure, bleeding and hormone treatment, bleeding and no hormone treatment, hormone treatment alone, excessive nausea, hormone treatment or excessive nausea, varicose veins, excessive weight gain, and X-rays. By far the greatest relative risks the questionnaire revealed were for women who had taken hormones in any of the categories mentioned. The authors wrote: "In this study we . . . found excessive nausea and exogenous hormone use during the index [studied] pregnancy to be high risks for testis cancer." Exogenous hormones are hormones introduced into the body rather than those the body manufactures itself.

The authors also factored into their study the incidence of undescended testicles, which since the late 1940s have been associated with testicular cancer. The reason for the association between cancer and undescended testicles is not clear, but the authors wanted to see if whatever factors caused a testicle to be undescended at birth might also be related to testicular cancer.

Combining all the elements, the Henderson paper concluded: "A major risk factor for testis cancer (and cryptorchidism) is a relative excess of certain hormones (estrogen and perhaps progesterone) at the time of testicular differentiation (7th week). The impact of these events, if any, on the subsequent expression of male characteristics must be subtle since fertility does not appear to be directly affected."

The paper also stated that estrogens in general had been shown in 1960 to cause cancer in certain strains of mice, and researcher John A. McLachlan had shown in 1975 that DES could produce incomplete genitalia development and undescended or improperly descended testicles in offspring born to pregnant animals injected with it.

John A. McLachlan, Ph.D., is a highly respected developmental toxicologist at the National Institute of Environmental Health Sciences in North Carolina. He works with animals to try to anticipate the effects of drugs when used in humans. In 1975 he and his colleagues published a paper showing that male offspring of pregnant rodents injected with DES developed cryptorchidism. The incidence of this same problem in DES sons was published about three years later. McLachlan's animal studies with DES were used prominently at all congressional hearings looking into the use of DES both for humans and as an animal food additive.

Recently one of eight DES-exposed mice in McLachlan's colony developed invasive seminal vesicle carcinosarcoma (cancer cells in the seminal vesicles, a part of the male reproductive system). In humans, invasive seminal vesicle carcinosarcoma is a rare form of testicular cancer. Three of the eight DES-exposed mice developed, among other abnormalities, interstitial cell tumors (tumors in between the cells in the testes). Neither of these types of growths appeared in the control mice used. And although some tumors are benign, all tumors have the capability to become cancerous.

McLachlan wrote, in the Herbst-Bern textbook where these animal findings were first reported: "Epididymal cysts were expected . . . but the finding of an invasive seminal vesicle carcinosarcoma was not." To eliminate the possibility of coincidence, the records were searched for the occurrence of this type of cancer cell in other rodents. "Spontaneous carcinomas of the male rodent accessory sex glands are rare," McLachlan stated. "The carcinosarcoma of the seminal vesicle seen in the [DES-exposed mouse] raises the possibility that these structures are potential targets."

In effect, based on these findings in animals, DES may have an impact on the wolffian duct remnants in males and the later development of testicular cancer, just as it has an effect on the müllerian duct remnants in females and the later development of clear-cell adenocarcinoma of the vagina.

McLachlan cautioned: "Although the changes observed in rodents after DES exposure may not appear in humans, experimental results from appropriate animal models can be informative." He pointed out that his laboratory found undescended testicles in animals three years before such a finding for humans was published and stated: "The possible relevance of animal models in the areas under discussion needs no further comment."

* * *

For several years after his graduation from law school twenty-seven-year-old attorney Craig A. Diamond worked for the Los Angeles firm of Haight, Dickson, Brown, & Bonesteel, which is in charge of the DES defense strategy for E. R. Squibb & Sons. Diamond himself helped defend many DES cases for Squibb.

In August 1980 Craig went to a physician, complaining of soreness and unusual development of his breasts. "The doctor told me to take two aspirins and 'Don't worry about it,'" recalled Craig. Three months later his urine "was the color of bourbon," and another physician diagnosed him as having four types of cancer cells in his right testicle, which was surgically removed.

After he had started working on the Squibb company's defense, Craig asked his mother whether she had used DES. "I was concerned more with my sister than with myself. I found out that she had not taken it with my sister but had taken it subsequently. Since my sister and I are the only surviving children, I didn't bother asking any further. Many months down the line, when I found out I was sick, I asked my mother, and found out that indeed she had taken it with me, and I just put two and two together."

Craig Diamond has filed a lawsuit against many DES manufacturers because he does not know which company manufactured the DES his mother took. He has hired his former adversary, plaintiffs' attorney Roman Silberfeld, who frequently represented women who were suing Squibb. "I had followed him around for so long that I knew he was competent, so I wouldn't mind having him represent me," Diamond said. He has also filed a medical malpractice suit against the physician who told him to take the aspirin for the discomfort in his breasts, which was apparently caused by the same cellular explosion that caused the testicular cancer.

There was a sigh as Craig Diamond paused to consider his anomalous position as an attorney who once defended a major drug company in DES suits and was now suing many of them because of his own DES exposure. "In retrospect, I don't feel bad for having done what I had done, nor do I have any bad feelings about my buddy [a friend in his former firm] doing what he has to do. I think it's a lawyer's responsibility to give his client the best defense possible. The people at Haight, Dickson have been spectacular throughout my illness—they couldn't be more supportive."

After his surgery and convalescence he resigned from the law firm. "I decided I was leaving Los Angeles. I had always wanted to live in the country, and once I had this life crisis, I figured this was as good a time as any." He now works for a small firm in Grass Valley, California, a community in the gold rush hills between Sacramento and Lake Tahoe, and handles a general range of legal concerns—real estate, wills, and personal matters. He said he is not opposed to working for insurance companies or defending companies against lawsuits.

"A life crisis," said Craig, "is when you think you're going to die. Every other crisis that anyone has, you either succeed or you fail—you can bounce back, or hurt, or whatever, but there's always tomorrow. But with something like this there's no tomorrow. So it comes down to living, and the quality of your life."

The quality of his life now, he said, "on the surface is fine. I still have a lot of tenderness and a lot of physical problems, but it's like having an axe over your head—you just never know when it's going to fall. If something irregular happens to me I'm going to have chemotherapy, and that's not something I look forward to—I watched my father go through chemotherapy. Most people get a cold and feel terrible. I have to be especially alert that it's a cold, that I'm not getting seriously sick again."

Craig has gotten fulfillment from his work, which has helped him balance the new adjustments he needs to make in his personal life. "I'm a very social person—always have been—and for a while I became very introspective, almost hermitlike. That lasted a couple of months, and now I'm stepping out. I don't particularly stay away from members of the opposite sex, though I'm very self-conscious about it at times physically. Not only do I have only one testicle but I have a scar that runs almost the length of my body" (the result of the lymph-node operation that searched for, but did not find, the spread of cancer). In 1982, Craig Diamond married, and his wife recently gave birth to a baby girl, Lacee.

But it is also a job just to keep healthy and whole. "I try to stay active and keep a good mental attitude, but sometimes it just doesn't work. It gets to be exhausting, for a person who's never really been sick, to have to live every day like this. I'm very, very tired of being sick and living right on the edge of the sword."

Although there has been no proven association between DES use by pregnant women and testicular cancer years later in their sons, one physician who believes that such a connection will eventually be made is Thomas Sansone, M.D., who removed the cancer-filled right testicle from Philadelphia plumber Francis X. Lawler on August 3, 1981. "In my speculative opinion," Sansone said, "DES will eventually be shown to be carcinogenic in men who were exposed *in utero*. DES will be shown to be responsible in part for the rise of testicular cancer."

The types of cancer that struck Frannie Lawler were seminoma and embryonal cell cancers. "Believe me, nothing embarrasses me now," Frannie Lawler said laughing. "I was a modest person at one time, but now I couldn't care less." The twenty-five-year-old Lawler, the father of a young son, has been told by his maternal aunt that his mother took DES during her pregnancy with him. His mother died in 1979 from bone cancer, having previously had breast cancer.

Curiously, the Lawlers' story begins with Susan, Frannie's wife, also born in 1956, who is a DES daughter. Her story was presented in more detail in the chapter on miscarriages. Susan Lawler had three miscarriages before giving birth to their son, Keith Ryan Lawler, on September 19, 1980.

After the baby's birth the Lawlers were living in a new house they had bought in the country. "I returned to work [as a supermarket clerk] eight weeks after the baby was born, and then I noticed that my husband had an abnormality—one testicle seemed different, harder." They noticed the difference in the right testicle in April or May of 1981. "I thought it was a strain, from moving or lifting something. In my work as a plumber I sometimes lift a hundred pounds or more," Frannie said. He went to the doctor at work, who said it was irregular but not abnormal.

"But it was getting bigger all the time, and I knew I'd have to do something. It scared the hell out of me! I don't like going to doctors." He speaks with the forcefulness and verbal jousts of the Philadelphia streets where he grew up, and talks about the experience with only a minimum of pauses and sighs.

He went to his family doctor, an osteopath, who said that an exploratory procedure was needed. At this point Frannie Lawler discovered that cutting, offhand remarks are not reserved only for women caught up in the medical process. "He said that the worst that can happen is that they'll pop a rubber ball in there [to replace the testicle]. Can you believe that? It came at me too fast. He didn't know me from Pete."

He then consulted two urologists, including Thomas Sansone, M.D., and on August 2 went into the hospital. The next day his right testicle and its attached cord were removed.

"When I woke up several hours later the doctor said the tumor showed two kinds of cancer, the seminoma and the embryonal, and because they were fearful it might have spread, they wanted to do another exploratory operation. I didn't think I had much choice. I felt I had to do it for the rest of my family." While he was listening to the doctors he was also watching the dozen balloons with "smiley faces" Susan had had delivered to him.

On August 10 he was back in surgery. "It was a retroperitoneal node dissection. They cut in around the chest, at my nipples, and cut down to my belly button, and off to the right, making a nice cute angle. They dissected my urinary tract, dissected fifteen lymph nodes, and removed my appendix while they were at it. The frozen sections they took came back fine, I'm clean as a whistle. They say the chances of a recurrence are ninety-five percent against."

The medical bill for the procedures came to $12,943, all of it covered by his insurance or hers. "Thank God for insurance," he added.

Although Frannie is still fertile, because one testicle remains, he has started to have retrograde ejaculation. "There's no difference in feeling with sex, but when I ejaculate, it goes into my bladder instead of out of my body, so I think it's going to be hard to have any more children."

They have come to terms with his situation in a loving and friendly way. "It's good to joke about it, no matter how it sounds," Frannie said. "Like maybe I should work in a Chinese restaurant and call myself One Hung Lo. All my friends know—it's not an embarrassment to me." But Susan said, "Sometimes it can go too far. When I was having D and C's because of my DES exposure, my friends would say that it was time for my 'dusting and cleaning.' But sometimes that kind of talk can cut you too."

His hospitalization became a new experience for her. "Frannie was always waiting outside the operating room for me, and now I was waiting for him. When the doctor told me it was cancer I was OK when I heard it, then when I went into the elevator I broke down and cried. At the hospital, before the second operation, we argued a lot. I was scared. I knew if they removed his other testicle, there would be no possibility of an erection. Should there be a second surgery, I wondered. That night I called the doctor up at home at eleven o'clock and talked to him for thirty minutes. It must have been a Monday night, because he had to turn the football game on the TV down so he could hear me."

His recuperation has given Frannie Lawler a new career—house husband. "I see things that most husbands don't get to see. I see the baby when he's sleeping, and crying, and his temper tantrums, and the crappiest diapers you'd ever want to see. I'm a good housewife—a good housewife and mother too."

In between his surgeries Frannie wrote his eleven-month-old son a letter. He had surrendered one testicle to cancer and didn't know what the future would bring.

> *To Master Keith Ryan Lawler, from Dad Lawler, Room 258. 1st class mail for a 1st class guy.*
>
> *I know it's been a long time since you and Dad have played and played bounce-bounce together, but that doesn't mean that I don't love you very much. It might be a little while until we can do really neat things together, so I thought I might write you this letter and try to explain what is going on. . . . Dad has what's called a tumor and had to go to the hospital and have it taken out. I went to the hospital the day we left you with Aunt Mary Ellen and Nanna, and I thought I would come home right after they took it out, but the doctor said it was a kind of cancer. Cancer is something that could hurt Dad, and he really doesn't know why or understand it at all, so I really don't expect you to understand it too much, even though you're the smartest little kid I know.*
>
> *Dad is going to try everything he knows to get this problem that has come between us out of the way so we can spend all the time in the world together.*
>
> *I just wanted to remind you that you are the most important little guy in my life, and I love you more than anything or anybody in the world, and I'll be home as soon as I can.*
>
>   *Love and Hugs,*
>   *Dad*
> *P.S.: Tell Mommy I miss her and love her, too, very much.*

11

MISCELLANEOUS MEDICAL PROBLEMS

One DES daughter I met had a partial vaginectomy at the age of nineteen to remove traces of adenosis. In the mid-1970s some doctors considered partial vaginectomies to be necessary measures in preventing cancer, which was then thought to spring from adenosis. Two years before that, she had had a cyst removed from her ovary. However, she didn't find out about the partial vaginectomy until she was twenty-five years old. Some partial vaginectomies have been known to affect the reproductive capacity of DES daughters. She does not know if this will happen to her, because she and her husband have not yet tried to start a family.

This woman is similar to many DES daughters in that she has a number of identifiable medical conditions that have been associated with DES, and although her physical health today is fine, she is unsure what the future will bring.

The 1981 paper by Arthur L. Herbst, M.D., and his colleagues, focusing on the fertility difficulties of DES daughters, also confirmed many other DES-related problems. The study, published in the December 15, 1981, issue of the *American Journal of Obstetrics and Gynecology*, showed that 32 percent of the DES daughters in the study had a shorter than normal menstrual cycle, compared to 15 percent of the unexposed women. And the mean duration of the menstrual flow for the DES daughters was 4.3 days, compared to 5 days for the unexposed. The reasons for the differences are not known.

Twenty-two DES daughters out of the total of 338 DES women had undergone laparoscopy, a delicate and sometimes painful microscopic examination of the abdominal and pelvic cavities. Only 4 of the 22 were regarded as normal. Eight of the women had pelvic inflammatory disease, 3 were anovulatory (had never ovulated), 2 others had a variety of cysts, and 3 had endometriosis. By contrast, 19 of the 298 unexposed women had undergone laparoscopy, and 9 were regarded as normal. Only one had pelvic inflammatory disease, 2 were anovulatory, 5 of the unexposed women had endometriosis, and none had cysts.

Perhaps reflecting the greater health-care concern of DES-exposed women, it was found that more of them had had a wider variety of surgical procedures than had nonexposed women. For example, 27 DES daughters had undergone curettage (the delicate and surgical cleansing of diseased tissue), compared to only 8 of the nonexposed. Sixteen DES women had had breast biopsies, compared to only 8 of the unexposed; and the DES women had undergone far more medical procedures, such as cervical conization (the removal of a cone-shaped piece of cervical tissue), cervical cerclage (a stitching of the cervix to strengthen it), hymenectomy (the excision of the hymen, the membrane at the front of the vaginal opening), tracheloplasty (repair of the uterine cervix), and hysterectomy (removal of the uterus), than had the unexposed women.

This woman doesn't know if she can have children because of her DES exposure or because of the possible harm done by the partial vaginectomy.

"My first period came late, when I was fourteen, and then it was always irregular. I had an ovarian cyst removed, and when I was nineteen I was told to come in because of adenosis, which I was told was a precancerous condition. The operation was pretty simple, done on an outpatient basis. [Later] I went to a gynecologist to be fitted for a diaphragm, and she said, 'Well, your vagina is very small because of the vaginectomy you've had.' "

We were sitting on the deck of the small hillside house she shares with her husband and their cats. As she recounted her experience her voice shook and she clenched her hand into an angry fist. "I was pretty shocked. I thought I had gone in for the removal of some cells, and five years later I felt as if my body had been deformed. I was *not* treated as an intelligent individual who was responsible for her own health! I was *not!*"

She had been a liberal arts major at a major university and later dropped out to open a plant shop. Then she saw a television program about the use of DES as a growth stimulant in animals headed for the dinner table and decided not to eat meat, because it might add to the level of DES she had had in her body since the day she was born.

"When I went to a doctor for birth control advice, she urged me to use the pill. I said I didn't want to, because they contain estrogens, and I was worried about the add-on effect with DES. She just said, 'Well, I'm the doctor, and I know best.' but I said, 'No, it's *my* body.' " It was while she was being measured for a diaphragm that she learned about the partial vaginectomy and its potential fertility implications.

Her husband has been with her through all of her DES-caused problems. "More than anything," he aid, "it creates a worry. Right now I'm not too excited about kids, but I might get upset later on if we can't have them. It hasn't come between us at all. Periodically she'll get into a fragile mood, just want to be by herself, but we all do that. She deals with it effectively, I think, but sometimes it makes her very, very angry."

Her DES experience has also influenced the choice of a career. "My interest was sparked by the news program. I realized there was much more to be learned about the relationship between food and the body. I think people should be responsible for their own bodies and should take an active part in their health care," she said.

She has also struggled to correct the imbalance in her relations with her parents that DES exposure has brought about. "I want to share with [my mother] all that I've learned about DES, all that I'm doing with the DES Action group, and the many positive effects this experience has had on my development. I know she feels real bad about it. She turns it off. I love her very much, and I don't blame my mother a bit, but she blames herself. But back then it was the mood of an era to take these wonder drugs."

"She was a joy to us from the moment she was born," her mother said by phone. "That has never changed. I do feel guilty when I read about all those things connected with DES. You have to. But when we feel that way, either she or I, we talk on the phone, ninety minutes or more, whenever it's necessary. We stay close that way." Her father was on the extension phone. "My wife feels it's better to talk like that on the phone than buy her a dress or a present. It helps them both. When I heard about all these DES things, there wasn't much I could do but love them both."

Other mothers and daughters have not worked out their DES bond so smoothly. One woman I talked to desperately needed to get her medical records to see if the fertility problems she was having could have been DES-related. She called her mother, "who has always been guilt-stricken about it," and asked her to go to the hospital. "She said she couldn't, she was getting her hair done. I asked my father, and he drove to the hospital. When they wouldn't give him the records, he threatened a lawsuit. They gave him the file. I am DES-exposed, and my mother and I never talk about it."

One DES mother hasn't been feeling too well lately, "and maybe it's because of DES—who knows?" She said she had recently been undergoing radiation treatment for uterine cancer, which resulted in a complete hysterectomy. The doctors told her they felt they had arrested the cancer, which showed up after she went through menopause. Her menopause "seemed to last forever," and in the last few months a tumor in her bladder had been found, which has also been surgically removed.

Other women not exposed to DES have had such problems. But is the DES she took a possible cause or contributing factor in her uterine cancer, bladder tumor, and difficult menopause? There are few studies of the first generation of DES women—the women who swallowed it, pill by pill, for seven or more months of their pregnancies. There is no proof that it is.

And no proof that it may not be.

Barbara Mullen, whose mother was unable to get pregnant for twelve years before taking DES, exemplifies the early age at which problems have appeared in some DES daughters. Just after she reached puberty it was dicovered that she had two ovarian cysts that would have to be removed. She also had adenosis.

"I was thirteen when we found out about what DES could do to people," Barbara said, speaking in soft and shy voice. "It's scary going to a gynecologist when you're fourteen, being the only girl on the block who knows what a gynecologist is. I didn't tell any of my friends about it, and I wonder about children of my own. I don't know how healthy I'm going to be. After the operation to remove the ovarian cyst the doctor told me I might not have children." At twenty-two Barbara is currently studying to be a dental hygienist at Pasadena City College and is preparing to be married.

Barbara's mother, Joy Mullen, noticed other problems early on in her pregnancy with Barbara, when she was taking DES as recommended by a fertility clinic. She started out weighing 117 pounds and in "almost no time at all" gained 68 pounds. "I know I didn't change my diet, but maybe that was the problem. Now I know about chicken and beef and how DES was used to fatten them up. I think that's what happened to me," Joy added. After Barbara was born in 1959 Joy noticed that "my back was filled with tiny cysts. No one could tell me the cause."

Many women have been hurt physically by DES, and some have been hurt mentally. This situation becomes much worse when a DES-exposed individual seeking medical help comes out of a doctor's office feeling more compromised than when she went in. Barbara Mullen was once examined by a gynecologist who sat in front of her "flipping through the pictures from my colposcope exam, singing 'You Ought to Be in Pictures.' He's done this for five years now and I'm sick of it. I keep going to him because he's an expert. But I avoid him when I can talk to his nurses for information."

The medical problems with DES have slowly evolved and been recognized over the last decade. It is still not clear whether the synthetic nature of the drug makes it more difficult for the body to metabolize it and get rid of it, when compared to natural estrogens. It is still not clear what effect normally produced body chemicals will have on cells that have already been influenced by DES. It is still not clear what effect other chemicals and substances, such as birth control pills, introduced into the body during the course of a lifetime, will have on those cells.

It is still not clear what will *happen* to people. For example, when this chapter was originally written, I had put the story of Laura Minor's early-life gynecological problems here. Between the time of our interview and the editing of this chapter Laura had become pregnant and then had a miscarriage, causing me to move her story to the section on miscarriages. Her situation is the one millions of DES-exposed people face: What will happen? When will it happen? How will I know?

12

PERSONAL IMPACT AND MEDICAL CALLOUSNESS

"After I got pregnant the first time we opened a bottle of champagne. The pregnancy lasted two months. We didn't dare celebrate the second one. The experience of finally having a successful pregnancy," the woman said, sighing, "almost ruined my marriage."

There is another dimension to DES exposure that has nothing to do with biopsies and Pap smears, testicle monitorings and self-exams. It is the hidden dimension of personal anguish, uncertainty, confusion, unhappiness, and, reportedly, divorce.

Many DES-exposed people have developed a sense of fatalism. They now know from their own experience that information about the drug and its impact changes over time. Concerns about the future must figure in decisions that are being made now and actions that are being taken today. Those concerns include anxiety about the impact of DES-related problems on wife and husband, mother and daughter, fear of sexual relations and social rejection— a whole bitter rainbow of distress. DES exposure does not have to be the end of the world, but to the DES population it just means they have to fight harder to stay even.

Many couples shared with me their experiences in relation to pregnancy but did not discuss the feelings of stress between them. They couldn't—having lived through it once was painful enough; reliving it again with a journalist was asking too much. But one couple was able to articulate the problems others had mentioned in bits and pieces and was willing to speak candidly. The wife is a thirty-year-old licensed health-care professional, who was born on April 18, 1951 in New York State. During a routine examination in 1975 her doctor said, "Ah, I see your mother took stilbestrol—you'd better start thinking about a family."

"I chose my career thinking family. I had the erroneous idea that medicine as a career would not allow me to be the type of mother I hoped to be. The experience at the time left me feeling somewhat defeated, empty." In addition to miscarrying her first pregnancy, she has also had infertility problems for most of her marriage. "I kept getting pregnant, but they wouldn't hold. I thought I was going crazy. I was beginning to believe I was having pseudopregnancies, like a dog. In fact, they were two-week gestational pregnancies."

Her first concern, after the doctor's suggestion that she start thinking about a family, was cancer. "There's a smell about a cancer patient, and you can see the pain, and you think, How can one live with such knowledge—that there is a cancerous growth consuming a vagina, or organs, or your body?" Her second concern was her husband, an upper-income professional, a man with whom she shares a love of sports and outdoor life but with whom she was unable to share her fears about the impact of DES.

"He was coldly analytical. He said, 'If you think you have cancer, go see a specialist.' That kind of attitude almost ended our marriage. He joined the DES Registry [one of the consumer groups] without telling me. He was afraid that if I read too much about it it would interfere with our attempts at getting pregnant."

But trying to get pregnant created its own problems. "We would have sex every month following the temperature charts [which determine the optimal moment for conception to take place]. If he didn't come home from his rugby practice right away, I'd get mad. 'What do you mean, you had a beer with the boys? I was waiting for you.' Here I was, freaking out like a dog in a pseudopregnancy. Your breasts get tender, you get this aura, this feeling," she said vehemently. "You can always cut out a cancerous part, but infertility is different. That's your life's dreams. But now I realized I wasn't in control. *I had no control over my own destiny.*" The situation, she added reflectively, caused "a lot of stress in my marriage."

She hesitated a moment before exploring the stresses they were under. "I'm sure I wasn't pleasant to be with. I was twenty-seven, healthy [but] my body was deteriorating. I hated everything I had to do to get pregnant—the tests, the monitoring, everything became intolerable. But the biggest threat was his lack of compassion regarding my bleeding, which would occur irregularly, anytime. Once I was driving back from Baltimore and I started bleeding. The next day I told him that it might indicate cancer. He didn't touch me. He said, 'If you think it's true, go see a doctor.' Because of this I really disliked him. Even now, if I have an emotional need he's not the one I turn to. When you need someone emotionally, it doesn't matter what they *think*. You learn not to grasp for them or expect them to come through."

Her husband acknowledged he is an analytical person, but he added some insight into a man's difficulty in understanding the frightening aspects these problems can create for women. "I can't see the bleeding, I can't feel it, I can't go into the bathroom with her. We were having emotional stresses on top of this." Then he added: "She is a very healthy person, she seems to be strong and healthy, but she can be fragile and dependent. Once she was scared of the dark at a cabin—she wouldn't go out because I had jokingly told her not to be afraid of the werewolves. She had tears in her eyes." His wife made him go with her with a flashlight.

For the first pregnancy, which lasted two months, they had opened the champagne. "We ignored it for the second one. We didn't want to invest the emotion; it was too precarious." What was also precarious was their life together. "Marriagewise, he was more concerned about the baby. He said, 'This might be the only baby we'll ever have, so everything's got to be perfect.' I'd have a cup of coffee and he'd say, 'How can you do this to *our* baby?' I had an emotional outburst—'*You never ask about ME!*' There was no more sex—he refused intercourse, all physical contact except for hugging. He was very protective, very supportive, but our whole life changed."

Her husband's response echoed his fears about the pregnancy for both his unborn child and his wife. "I didn't want to blow it. We'd been through so much, I simply made a decision I didn't want to take any chances. The women's groups and her doctors were saying there was no problem with sex during pregnancy, but I read in a medical journal that there might be a problem. I just made a decision we wouldn't take any chances. I made up my mind that's what we'd do, and we did it. I never yelled at her for coffee or a beer, I'd just made a remark."

The weight of this frank discussion was causing her to shut her pale blue eyes periodically. Candor carries its own price. And she also was thinking about, hoping for, her baby's birth.

Shortly after we spoke their child was born, a healthy baby, and with

it the hope that the couple's marital stresses might be over. In a
note after our interview, however, the woman wrote: "The ordeal revealed some character traits that will always be a part of our marriage,
something we always will have to deal with and something that
will always preclude an emotional commitment and exposure on my
part."

Another young couple talked about their sexual relations this way:
"I'm always afraid I'm going to hurt her," the husband said. "I've got a
mental block against it. And after sex she does seem to have a problem,
she does hurt. Does abstinence create stress? Oh, yeah. We are definitely on a low-to-nonexistent [sexual] level."

His wife of more than a dozen years undergoes frequent biopsies, has
a history of ovarian tumors, and has had a fallopian tube removed. She
added: "I'm afraid making love is going to hurt, and if it does, I don't
want him to know it. In the last two years it has gotten more and more
painful. There are lots of things other women can give him—kids, sex,
earn money. I can't. I'm sick a lot. I have a lot of infections. I've got to
stay home and rest—"

Her husband cut in, "When she's sick she reads novels. You know
the last time I read a novel? It was years ago. I can't be sick, because of
her."

She added softly, "It's the little luxuries I have, when I'm sick, reading . . ."

DES-related infertility creates many kinds of sexual anxieties and
varying stress reactions. One couple tried for years to get pregnant,
blaming the wife's confirmed DES exposure for their failure. Then
clinical tests showed that her fertility had not been affected, but his
DES exposure, about which they had known for years, had apparently
caused an unusually low sperm count. The woman described that moment: "When my husband found out about what his DES exposure
meant, he stopped sleeping with me completely for nearly half a year,"
she said. "He got completely depressed. He wouldn't touch me. Later,
when we found out that some surgery might correct the problem he
has, a low sperm count, he became like a bull in spring. We are trying
to get pregnant now."

Another man was deeply anxious throughout his adolescence about
the moment of his first sexual experience and how women would react
to him sexually. He has microphallus. "I was afraid with women, I delayed having sex because of the fear. Would they laugh at me? Would

they humiliate me? Would I be sexually adequate? These thoughts haunted me for years. Finally I met a girl from down the street who was very sexually aggressive, and it happened so fast there were no questions asked."

The man is now married, has two children, and his wife protectively said that there were "no problems, none, during intercourse."

But when she was not near us he said: "My penis is okay during erection, and obviously, with kids, we know there's no problem with fertility. But it sometimes hurts during intercourse, and she asks me if it's okay. I don't like it that she has to ask, I don't like that extra burden being on her."

He explains that as a young man he was "embarrassed in front of the other boys. When I went to the YMCA for a steam bath I was the only one wrapped in a towel around my waist or wearing shorts. But that only drew more attention to it. The solution was that I stopped going to the YMCA. In the Army I continued this embarrassment—I tried to shower or use the locker room when no one else was there. It affects everything you do."

Fears about sexual attractiveness and performance can also affect choice of sexual partners. One woman I spoke with has chosen a gay relationship. She and her friend own a home together which they are fixing up. Now in her thirties, she has known of her DES exposure for more than a decade.

"I was involved with a man once, for more than a year, but never had sex with him. I was afraid of myself, afraid of what he might say if he knew about DES. It became a stigma. I was afraid to tell him, and I was afraid to establish any kind of close emotional relationship with him because I was afraid he would ultimately reject me. I don't know if I'm fertile, but during the years I was dating men I never used any birth control measures, and I never got pregnant. Maybe it was luck or maybe I'm infertile."

As she became more involved with the routine of complete examinations every six months, she found herself with an increasing desire to share her problems with "someone, anyone. It's easier to talk to another woman than it is to talk to a man. At least it is for me."

She and her friend have been together for several years. "I do get a lot of support from her; it's support I needed, and need."

I asked her if she thought she would have chosen a gay life-style if she were not DES-exposed. Her eyes became misty, and she looked up with pain and longing. She shrugged.

*   *   *

The DES experience has also alienated women from their doctors and raised problems for those mothers trying to get proof of their DES exposure so they can prepare their prepubescent daughters.

Sally Abramson, of Chevy Chase, Maryland, wanted to find the doctor who had given her pills during pregnancy. She now suspects those pills were DES. "I tried to find the doctor after all these years, but he had retired to the South. I tracked him down to some small town and asked him over the phone. He denied it. But I didn't believe him—the word 'stilbestrol' stuck in my mind. I called the hospital where I'd been treated and found a sympathetic records worker. *She* was a DES daughter. She pulled my records—I think it may have been a violation of hospital policy at the time—and sent them to my present Ob-Gyn. Sure enough, there on the records was written 'stilbestrol.' My daughter so far is fine, thank God. She was a teenager then, and now she's in college, but I don't think that's the way for doctors to behave."

Beryl Rothman, of Rockville, Maryland, said her doctor told her "he gave it routinely to all his patients, whether they'd been pregnant before or not, whether they were having problems or not. He told me he gave it to 'all his girls.' He told me he did it for 'insurance.' That means there must be thousands of boys and girls out there who are DES babies and may not know it."

That raised another problem for her, as it does for other DES mothers—having her daughter examined. "I didn't want to go to just any doctor. My daughter was fourteen. I wanted a pediatric gynecologist, someone who specialized in young girls. I started to shop around. I talked to the doctors first, before making an appointment. Several told me there would be no problem with an exam, but I felt there might be, because of her age. When I found one who sounded right, I waited a month before I could get an appointment. But I still hadn't told my daughter why she was going to be examined.

"I made a couple of mistakes. I didn't tell her myself, and I underestimated her ability to understand. I should have given her more credit. Maybe I didn't have enough faith in *my* ability to deal with it. I'm grateful there's no malignancy, but who needed it? It's added an extra dimension to my life, though: I've never been a statistic before."

Beryl had a second daughter in 1970, "who may be one of the last children exposed to DES. She has not had her first period yet, so we have the whole routine to go through with her. I'm not going to make the same mistake twice, of not telling her ahead of time."

Her oldest daughter, Stephanie, is now a ninth-grade student. When I spoke with her, she had to ask her mother how DES had affected her: an incomplete cervical hood and adenosis. She was two days away from her fifteenth birthday.

"At first I felt a little sorry for myself," Stephanie said. "I was angry, and a little scared. I read *DES Daughter* [a personal account by Joyce Bichler], and I worried about getting cancer or something like that. But I'm glad there's nothing really wrong with me. I'm sure I must have friends who are also DES children, but I don't know if they know themselves. It's not something you go up and ask somebody about."

In 1971 Mary Patton, of Alexandria, Virginia, learned during a routine gynecological examination of the new reports linking cancer to DES daughters. Mary's daughter Nola was then six years old. The doctor advised waiting a few years before having Nola examined. When Nola turned fourteen she was examined by a DES specialist, who found no problems, although her mother did not tell her why she was being examined. "I didn't want to worry her," Mary Patton said.

Recently, shortly after her sixteenth birthday, Mrs. Patton did tell Nola. "I was scared, because I thought it would automatically mean I'd have cancer," the eleventh-grade student said. "But now I don't worry about it much. Now and then I think about it, yeah, but I don't talk to my friends about it at school, because it's very personal," she added shyly.

One DES mother ran into a farce with her former physician, which fortunately has not resulted in any harm to her or her son. Claire Smith (now of Bethesda, Maryland) was living in Urbana, Illinois, when her doctor gave her DES pills. Her son, born in 1949, has no problems, she said. In an attempt to find out whether she had been given DES, she wrote to her former doctor, asking him to check his records, and in his reply he suggested that she keep him advised of any problems affecting her *daughter*. When she wrote back and said that she had had a son, he double-checked his files, which stated that she had given birth to a girl, and reconfirmed that he had given Claire DES.

Claire Smith was angered not only because the doctor had gotten the sex of her child wrong but also because she had been given the pills in her first pregnancy, and therefore could never have had a previous miscarriage.

*　　*　　*

There are countless examples of the hostility, callousness, or indifference with which the medical profession has responded to women's search for information.

Linda Marks, an attorney in Washington, D.C., was born in 1956. When she was just eighteen she was diagnosed as having adenosis and a cockscomb cervix. Later when she was twenty-three, she found she had severe dysplasia. "I was one of [the doctor's] first DES patients, and at first he was very understanding. Then I quickly realized that I was also a test case, with other doctors coming in to look. Suddenly I would hear strangers saying, 'Oh, look at that,' and I didn't know what they were looking at or what it meant. On another occasion a doctor was taking a picture, using a colposcope [the high-powered microscope that is sometimes favored with DES daughters because it can detect microscopic cellular changes]. The doctor suddenly said, 'Smile,' and I said, 'Doctor, I don't think that's what you're taking a picture of.'" Linda is aware the doctor may have been exercising what he thought were "examining-table manners," but she feels the remark was inappropriate and insensitive.

"In the early days all you read about was the association between DES and cancer. *There was no other information available!* It bothers me that doctors I meet now coming out of medical school seem to know so little about DES."

One physician, who had just graduated from a reputable east coast medical school told me that she had been given lectures on DES and its implications for women. She saw these talks as a sign of improved attitudes in the medical community. When I asked her what she had been told about the exposure of DES sons, she said with astonishment, "What about men? They weren't exposed."

Jo Ellen Morell tried to find out from physicians at a leading medical center about the extent of damage caused by her apparent DES exposure. Although she has not been able to prove that her mother took DES, Jo Ellen has typical signs of a DES daughter: adenosis and a hooded cervix. She described her experience during an examination at the center. "A doctor started to ask me all kinds of weird questions about how many times I'd had intercourse, how long it took me to have an orgasm, how many partners I'd had, and so on. As someone who is fairly naïve and innocent, I was bowled over. I wanted to find out about DES! About the chances of cancer! More than a year later someone else at the clinic told me I was part of a study—but I couldn't find out what that kind of a study had been for. They just wrote me off as someone who wouldn't understand them."

Jo Ellen was born on November 9, 1950, in Columbia, South Carolina, and was married in September 1981. She and her husband have not yet tried to have children, "but I would certainly want that option. It is pretty aggravating to think that something that happened thirty-one years ago would prevent that."

She was first warned about the possibilities of cancer, but what has actually hurt her the most is the treatment she received during the medical process. "I had my first gynecological exam ever in 1974 in Boston. The doctor noticed adenosis and a hooded cervix. All he talked about was cancer. He scared the tar out of me. I went to another doctor for a second opinion, and he said he'd wait six months before trying to find out the extent of my problem."

Since the first doctor had discussed only cancer, Jo Ellen was shocked when the second physician casually advised her to wait half a year before considering what to do. She started to cry, and the physician told her the crying was proof that she was emotionally unstable. "I said he would be upset too if he thought he had cancer of the genitals. When I did go back six months later, his colleagues kept walking in and out of the examining room, treating me like a piece of meat."

She moved to a suburb of Washington, D.C., but the change of locale did not end the humiliating experiences. "After I'd been biopsied and colposcoped, the doctor left the room while I was on the examining table, with my feet in the stirrups, facing the door. *He left the door open.* The people walking in the hall could have a good look-see." She asked the nurse not only to close the door but also to tell her what her limitations were regarding such things as tampons and hygiene. "She went into the hallway, *leaving the door open,* and asked him. He sort of shrugged and said, 'Tell her she can do it anytime.' I was mortified. I wasn't talking about sex. I wanted to slink out of there."

But not all doctors have been so insensitive or indifferent, Jo Ellen Morrell pointed out. "My current doctor once told me that I only had to come back once a year for exams. Later he wrote me a letter in his own handwriting saying that the research had changed and that I should now come back twice a year. I appreciated that," she said.

Joy Bender Heasley's problems with the medical establishment were hardly limited to her unwitting participation in a sex survey. "It's embarrassing and humiliating enough having to 'open wide' [undergo a pelvic exam] every six months, but I was not prepared for this. I was in a doctor's office having a colposcopic exam. A speculum was in my vagina when the light in the colposcope went out. The bulb had gone dead. The doctor left the office to call for the hospital maintenance man to change the bulb, *without covering me up!* The guy came in with the bulb, wearing his maintenance man's uniform, and changed the bulb, just like it was in the hallway! I marvel sometimes at the insensitivity of the medical profession."

Joy Heasley and her husband, Alfred Robert (Butch) Heasley, of Portsmouth, Virginia, have endured four years of trying to get pregnant, have gone through an ectopic pregnancy in 1981, and recently were disheartened by a pregnancy that failed after eight weeks. Their greatest worry is whether they can ever have children.

"If I manage to get pregnant again, what will happen?" Joy asked. "Will I be able to carry to term? There are a lot of kids out there who need homes. The paper work has begun for adoption. We're considering miscrosurgery to repair the tube damaged by the ectopic [pregnancy]. Our lives must go on with or without children."

Butch Heasley added: "I'm the only son of an only son of an only son. I think my [relatives] would be upset if we adopted. But I don't care. I've always wanted a kid of our own."

"I have a very supportive husband," Joy said, admiringly. "I couldn't go through this without him."

The stresses on DES-exposed individuals are not only physical and emotional but economic as well. Rachel Mary Wetherill, thirty, keeps her job with the federal government, in its insurance and health-care program, partially because of the medical expenses she incurs as a result of her DES exposure. "I have medical expenses that run about a hundred and thirty dollars every six months. Keeping this job is stability. Recently I had a chance at another job, working as a photographer for a small newspaper at half the salary. I would have loved it, but I'm afraid to be without health insurance, in case there is a major expense in the future."

Rachel was born in Chicago on November 16, 1951. Twelve *days* later her mother noticed a small growth on Rachel's vagina. Rachel's mother, Phyllis, had never been pregnant before, could not have had any miscarriage problems before, and therefore would probably never have taken DES if she hadn't gone to a major medical center for the best medical care she could find. "As of today I have adenosis, and had one vaginal cyst removed in 1979 and another removed in 1980," Rachel explained. "There are some new cysts now, but I am reluctant to go back into the hospital. Every time my period is early, or late, heavy or light, I think about what it could mean. It's the first question on my mind."

When Rachel was seventeen, in 1969, before she had any knowledge of DES and before any relevant medical reports had been published, a gynecologist said, " 'There's something wrong, there are bumps in there,' and advised me against using the pill for birth control."

Six years later her family received a letter from the hospital where she had been born, suggesting she get a checkup. "I heard my parents talking about a 'serious illness.' I assumed it was about my sister, it couldn't possibly be me—what could possibly be wrong with me?" When Rachel was examined she learned of her exposure and its possible consequences. "Every time a biopsy report comes back, it could be malignant. I see myself as a healthy person, physically healthy, but sometimes there is a struggle. If you see adenosis as an overwhelming problem, then that will make it worse. I try to keep an optimistic outlook on life."

She lives in a small frame house in rural Virginia, working as a rural letter carrier for the post office. We sat on her front porch and talked. She said she turned down the job at the local paper because it didn't have any health insurance. The hundred and thirty dollars she spends for exams every six months was not the determining factor so much as the financial obligations that might be incurred if her medical problems grow worse.

"There are lots of things I can't do because of DES, because I must stay near a doctor's office. I can't go out and hitchhike to Mexico, I can't do carefree things I did before 1975 [when she learned of her DES exposure]. I don't have that freedom now. I have some responsibility to myself, not to take chances, to stay near a major medical institution."

Like other women, she has found herself angered and humiliated by flippant remarks during examinations. "They treat you like a piece of meat, moving interns in and out to look at you, then telling you you're okay. After the biopsies, which they keep telling you are so important, you have to wait two or three weeks to find out the results. You keep thinking, Will I still be healthy? And the biopsies *hurt*; afterward you feel like you've been raped."

She is involved with lawsuits against the University of Chicago, where her mother received the DES, and against Eli Lilly & Company.

Rachel's mother was one of the three women who sued the University of Chicago for battery, claiming that they were not aware they were being given DES. In an out-of-court settlement in early 1982 the school agreed to pay the women $225,000, while not admitting guilt. "In part, I think the lawsuits will make people think twice before they do something like this again," Rachel said. "I was tremendously scared when I first found out about this. Now I'm just angry."

During one interview I found myself talking to a woman who had known of her own DES exposure for some time, but had just learned of the potential consequences of her husband's DES exposure. Now she understood why they had been having problems getting pregnant, and now she was terrified that they never would.

Her emotions were absolutely on the surface, unmoderated by time, information, or friends. As we sat in the kitchen area of her elegant Manhattan loft, it seemed to me that the raw feelings she was expressing must be identical to those felt by so many others at the very moment of their personal crisis.

"I have this fantasy, if I ever have a baby, I don't want my mother here. I won't tell her. She told me once, long ago, she'd taken DES for varicose veins when she was pregnant with me, but when I started having problems getting pregnant, she denied ever saying that. Yet I remember everything about that moment, the street corner we were on, it was Sixty-fourth Street, and the way the sun was slanting through the buildings. But she denied ever saying it—*my own mother*—and then that created so much guilt in her that she later said, 'You'd be a rotten mother anyway—you can't have a baby in this house, a baby shouldn't live in a loft.' "

She paused to light a cigarette. Smoking was a habit she had acquired with a self-destructive vengeance as the impact of her DES exposure became known. She kept it up for several months until her hard cigarette cough caused her to strain two ribs.

"I called the doctor's office in Iowa, but he had died and the records had been burned, *they said,* so I have no sure way of knowing, but I'll remember forever what [my mother] said and how she said it. I've had unexplained medical problems all my life; when I was eleven they said I had an aorta problem, as well as difficulty in getting food to move through the bowels and be excreted. That's going away now. I have a very small vagina, I had to cut tampons in half, coat them with ointment—but I grew out of that at age twenty-four. It's made me *enraged* with my parents. It's put my father between a rock and a hard-place—

he wants to help me, but he doesn't want to hurt my mother. Why me? Why am I the one to go through this, without help? No one talks about it—my husband is also DES-exposed, but he won't talk about it. His mother told him once and then denied it years later. It all just makes me so mad.

"It's hard for my mother to relate to what I'm doing. She got married and pregnant, and that's all she did. She calls here and all she can talk about is grandchildren. *I don't count!* She doesn't come here anymore—there aren't any grandchildren for her to play with."

Another pause, another cigarette, a hand that flicks across wet-rimmed eyes.

"I'm jealous of my sisters who have kids. My husband called me on the phone when I was out of town to say my sister was pregnant again and I burst out crying. I called my father to say I felt cheated and hurt, and I'm sure he feels the same way, but all he said was, 'You'll work it out.' I did, I worked it out, I cried all through a flight to Houston. You know the movie *Arthur?* How funny it is? I cried all through it.

"I come to terms with it by burying it. I'm sure some of it will resurface, especially if it turns out I can never have children. It's not inevitable that I won't have children, but it's going to be hard. The world knows me as a busy, noisy career broad, but I was raised to be a mother and I don't want to give that up. Every move that I make in my career is now tailored to having children. I made sure my new office was big enough for a crib in case I'm still breast-feeding. I turned down another job because I know they wouldn't give me maternity leave.

"*I feel betrayed!* I can't quite believe that at any time anyone thought that any pills during pregnancy were any good. I would be less emotional if I could get some facts, but my mother denies it, and my doctor just wants to keep me calm and won't tell me anything. I have a friend with the same problem. She's going through fertility procedures. Every day her husband masturbates into a vial and she rushes uptown to a clinic, and thirty minutes later the doctor injects it way up into her fallopian tubes, because the lining of her endometrium can't hold an egg. This has been going on for a year and a half, and I'm scared I'll have to go through that too."

At one point I said that even during the very early days of DES use there were important studies showing that it had no effect on preventing miscarriages. She said, as if she'd been shot, "*Oh, no! Don't take that away from me! Don't tell me I didn't have to go through this!*"

The woman later expressed some compassion for her parents, but with the rawness of her emotions at that extraordinary meeting, with the power of her feelings, she had presented an almost archaeological view of the force that lies beneath the surface of the lives of some of the DES-exposed people.

13

PSYCHOLOGICAL TESTS AND BRAIN WAVE MANIPULATION

There is another, darker effect of psychological import that DES may have had, one that is extremely difficult to research: that as DES influenced a fetus *in utero*, it may have determined how the person would act and respond after birth and throughout life.

This should have come as no surprise. DES is a potent sex hormone. When Sir Charles Dodds injected old male chickens with DES he feminized them: he changed the ways their bodies responded. Implanted with DES, the tough old birds became tender, juicier; that had been the whole idea. When DES was being synthesized in Dodds's London laboratories, the lightweight materials flew all around the room, and the workmen in the labs developed large breasts. They too were feminized.

The development of breasts in men or the tenderization of chickens, however, is only the external expression of a change in the body's delicate hormonal system. DES entered the body and told the brain, or the hormonal controlling factors, to act in a certain way, and when that happened, those workmen developed breasts. DES changed the way the chemicals in the body acted.

June Machover Reinisch is an associate professor with a Ph.D. in the Psychology Department of Rutgers University. Her small, cluttered office overlooks a field that blooms lushly in the spring. For more than a decade she has been interested in "the long-term effects of prenatal events. Anything that affects the central nervous system is a 'flavorer' of personality," she said. "Colas, cigarettes, alcohol, whatever. Everything a mother experiences—food, or drink, or emotions—could have an impact before birth on one's personal and physical development."

She talks quickly and decisively, taking a book down from a shelf to check a reference or spinning around in the orange-cushioned chair to make a point.

"Human beings are not programmed for behavior, they are not really programmable. The human organism is the most flexible of all animals. We can fly, swim, walk, and are able to live comfortably outside of our ecological niche."

Several years ago she decided to see if DES had made an impact on the personalities of children born to women who had taken it. A study published in 1973 by I. D. Yalom and others had looked at the same question, studying nondiabetic sons of diabetic mothers who had been given DES at a Boston clinic. The Yalom study had concluded that the DES offspring of diabetic mothers were less aggressive, less assertive, had less athletic skill and grace, and performed less well on certain mental tests than unexposed controls.

Reinisch and William G. Karow, M.D., criticized the Yalom paper in a 1977 article in the *Archives of Sexual Behavior*. They raised questions about the relationship of dosage and timing of dosage to the final conclusions. They said the authors had not taken into account the potential impact of progestins—hormones that were also given as pregnancy supports—as well as the impact that drugs used to treat diabetes could have had on the fetus. And they agreed with a statement in the Yalom paper that some endocrine disorder in the diabetic women might have had an impact on the fetus. Still, Reinisch and Karow found the Yalom conclusions interesting, because they paralleled findings in animal research, which showed that estrogens could "feminize" the behavior of test animals.

In order to pursue the subject of the lifelong impact DES might have had on developing fetuses, without falling into the quagmire of confusing DES impact with the impact of other drugs, Reinisch designed a test that is classically elegant in scientific terms. She used only DES daughters and compared them with their own sisters who had not been exposed to the drug. There were 16 young women in the DES group and 16 sisters in the unexposed group. The total mean dosage of DES given to mothers of the DES-exposed sisters was 6,119 milligrams. (By way of comparison, the total mean dosage of DES given to women at the University of Chicago was 12,031 milligrams, and the total mean dosage of DES given to mothers of women in the DESAD project was 4,190 milligrams.) Reinisch's findings were precise, and they have been widely accepted: DES daughters in her study were more group-oriented and group-dependent than their nonexposed sisters.

In one of our conversations Reinisch explained the findings, which were published in the April 7, 1977, issue of *Nature* magazine. "DES kids do things with a group, with other people. They seem to have more friends than the control group. They seem to be more joiners. They work well with other people, they are not passive but want to be with other people; they would choose to work on a project with a group rather than choose to work alone."

The women in her group were tested on the standard Wechsler intelligence and Cattell personality tests. On most questions there was no significant difference in responses between the DES-exposed women and their unexposed sisters. However, there was a significant difference in response on two questions on the Cattell personality test. In both cases the responses of the DES-exposed people leaned significantly toward the side of group orientation and group dependence, Reinisch said.

In her *Nature* paper DES-exposed women were not the only ones studied. Reinisch also examined the effects of natural progestins and discovered that the progestin-exposed offspring also had significant personality differences when compared to their own unexposed sisters, as well as when compared to the DES group. "Significant differences between the [progestin] and [DES] treatment groups were found on five personality factors: [Progestin] group subjects were significantly more independent, sensitive, individualistic, self-assured and self-sufficient than the exposed offspring of [DES] group, while the [DES] group subjects were more group-oriented and group-dependent."

In our interview Reinisch added: "A DES-exposed person could be a loner, but less of a loner compared to a sibling. That's what I mean by a *flavorer* of personality. He or she would be a better team player than a nonexposed sibling, maybe a better account executive or committee member. DES kids tend to be more freely expressive [of their emotions], more active in groups, and less critical of others than their nonexposed siblings."

Reinisch hastened to point out again and again that DES was acting as a flavorer of *some* personality traits that are measured on standard tests. DES kids did not score differently on twelve other personality aspects on one test or show any significant difference in intelligence scores when measured on another test. "With a small sample, finding something that is statistically significant is more meaningful than use of a larger sample," she said. "DES is only one flavorer of personality, or temperament." Therefore "the hormones a mother takes during pregnancy do have some lifelong influence on the psychological development of their offspring," she concluded.

Across the country, in Los Angeles, a young researcher named Melissa Hines received her Doctor of Philosophy degree in psychology from UCLA in 1981. She wrote her thesis on DES-exposed people and brain lateralization, which she explained to me this way as we sat in her laboratory in UCLA's sprawling medical center: "The brain has two hemispheres, and each seems specialized for certain cognitive functions. In most people the left hemisphere excels at verbal functions, the right hemisphere in spatial functions. But this differs from person to person, and therefore you can get a measure of the strength of lateralization by separating sensory input to the two hemispheres."

Hines wanted to see if DES had had an effect on the sexual differentiation of the human brain. Like Reinisch, she chose women with confirmed DES exposure who also had sisters who were unexposed. Between July of 1979 and August of 1980 she tested the 16 pairs of women in her study, who had been chosen after a record-review search of more than 900 DES women in clinics at UCLA and Stanford University.

She tested the women on two types of tests: auditory (sound) stimulation and visual stimulation. "For these types of tests," she explained, "there is a scale of responses. Males tend to score toward one end of the scale, and females tend to score toward the other end." Between those two poles is the field on which most people's responses are measured. Her conclusions are that "DES-exposed women showed greater lateralization than their unexposed sisters. The DES-exposed women had responses that were more toward the masculine distribution than their unexposed siblings."

She said that "only in terms of their responses on these measurements, DES women tend to respond more like men to auditory and visual stimuli. These are not *abnormal* patterns. And the distribution for males and females in general overlap, so even though the responses for the DES group are more toward the masculine distribution, they are still well within the range of normal female responses." But they respond differently when compared to their nonexposed sisters.

I asked Hines what this meant in a practical sense. "We don't yet know exactly what this means in the real world," she said. "Based on cognitive and personality tests, it apparently means nothing that should have an influence on their day-to-day lives. But it is of great scientific interest because we are learning how sexes differentiate. And this provides a link between animal and human research."

In another interesting study Richard C. Pillard, M.D., associate professor of psychiatry at the Boston University School of Medicine, studied a small group of 16 adult males to measure the effects DES exposure had on their sexual preference. His control group consisted of 50 heterosexual men and 50 homosexual men, none of whom had been exposed to DES during pregnancy.

A questionnaire asked questions about sexual behavior and fantasies. Then Pillard administered several tests of masculinity/femininity, using such questions as "I prefer adventure stories to romance stories." He pointed out that "boys tend to prefer adventure stories, and girls prefer romances. The implication would be that if you found that the DES boys had very high femininity scores on tests like that, you would conclude that DES had feminized them." The findings, however, proved unremarkable in terms of sexual differentiation. The DES subjects had masculinity scores and sexual behavior just like those of nonexposed males.

Pillard added that he does not know to what degree, if at all, DES might have influenced the sexual preferences of some sons. "But I think it's not a settled question yet. Most of the people who were exposed to DES are clearly heterosexual. If there is an increase in the percent of gay men, it's a small increase."

Pillard wanted to continue examining that question and proposed a three-year study to look at the sexual orientation of DES sons. His request for $350,000 in government funds was turned down in the spring of 1981.

It is possible that this line of inquiry is facing hard times. The sheer number of people necessary to do a precise survey is staggering. In order to find the 16 sets of sisters for her survey Reinisch had to sift through 600 medical charts; Melissa Hines found her 16 pairs of sisters after reviewing 900 charts. At the same time, the subject is personally disturbing to many people who are otherwise eager to learn all they can about

DES and the impact of DES exposure. It is not easy to face the idea that one's very personality, the traits that distinguish one person from another, may have been subtly influenced before birth. And, unlike the compelling need to know precisely what the health risks are for a DES-exposed son or daughter, there may not be the same compelling need to know in what way one's personality has been altered by DES.

14

DES USE AS A "MORNING-AFTER" PILL

Maybe you didn't just have to want a baby to get DES. Maybe you just had to fear you were accidentally pregnant and went to a doctor or health clinic for what has become known as a "morning-after" pill.

Times change. By the 1960s the baby boom was over. The birth rate in the 1950s had stayed at about 25 babies born for every thousand people annually, but in 1960 it was down to 23.7 per thousand, and by 1965 it had fallen to 19.4, exactly the same rate it had been in 1940. National goals and ambitions were different; adults were more involved with their own lives and careers outside marriage. In the 1960s there were fewer marriages and more divorces than there had been in the 1950s, and people frequently talked about postponing marriage or children until their own educations were completed and their careers were launched.

An aspect of this was the so-called sexual revolution. People—single and married—were increasingly interested in choosing the degree and intensity of their own sexual activity and in deciding for themselves exactly when (or if) they wanted to have children, rather than worrying about conception taking place as an inevitable result of intercourse. The birth control pill was widely heralded as an agent of this change, although many conservative medical people then and now protested its use on the grounds of unproven safety and potential side effects. Birth control devices, such as the intrauterine device (IUD) or vaginal diaphragm (which had been available for more than fifty years), became increasingly popular protective devices for women, and manufacturers of condoms brought out a wide variety of new styles and shapes.

DES was there too in the cultural and national surge to prevent pregnancies—just as it had once been there to prevent miscarriages. Once again its use seemed to have a social benefit: it was cheap, powerful, could be taken in pill form, and it was available.

Chemically, DES works in people as it did in Charles Dodds's 1938 experiments with rabbits and rats: it prevents conception from taking place by causing the female eggs to "disintegrate." When used this way DES is actually a series of morning-after pills—two 25-milligram tablets each day for five days. The daily dose of DES when used as a morning-after pill is about five hundred times the amount of estrogen the body naturally produces. The 25-milligram pill recommended as a morning-after pill was also one of the strengths made by companies catering to the antimiscarriage market, which was, theoretically, eliminated in 1971 when the FDA contraindicated DES during pregnancy.

If nature abhors a vacuum, think of what some drug companies must have felt when they perceived customers who had a need that wasn't being met. Especially if, after 1971, they had supplies of DES on hand that they could no longer freely market for pregnancy use.

The Food and Drug Administration prides itself on not interfering with the practice of medicine; it merely approves drugs and drug products for certain specified uses. If a doctor then chooses to use a product for an unapproved use, that is his choice, and neither the FDA nor any other agency stands in his way. Unlike its approved use in preventing miscarriages, however, DES has never been approved for use as a morning-after pill, although a good deal of confusion exists on this point. In fact, a physician today would be within his legal rights in prescribing DES as a morning-after pill, and it is still widely used at birth control clinics around the country, according to physicians I interviewed. Moreover, several of them said that if a woman got pregnant after using DES this way, abortion might be suggested as an option, since all fetuses exposed to DES run the same risk of harm that we have seen documented for DES-exposed offspring.

In 1971, shortly before the Herbst, Ulfelder, Poskanzer paper on cancer was published, the *New England Journal of Medicine* published an article based on research at the University of Michigan, claiming that a study of 1,000 women had proven DES to be an absolutely effective morning-after pill. That was a retrospective study, which means women were located who had taken the drug previously, sometimes as much as a year or more earlier, and interviewed about their experiences. Among other things, such a study proves that DES was being used in its unapproved form as a postcoital contraceptive in the late 1960s.

When Herbst testified on Capitol Hill later in 1971 regarding the association between DES and cancer, he stated: "We do not have enough data or knowledge at the present time to say what the smallest dose or the shortest duration of exposure to this drug is that could cause trouble."

In 1972 an official from the National Institutes of Health stated that DES was being used at most university health clinics around the country as a morning-after pill. Because of the recent association between DES and cancer, and its widespread use in the agricultural industry, there was considerable concern about the usage of such a powerful drug in such large quantities. According to Sidney M. Wolfe, M.D., head of the consumer-oriented Health Research Group, total sales of DES increased in 1972, the year after it was banned for pregnancy use. Some DES was being legitimately used for postmenopausal replacement therapy, some of it was being used to fight cancer of the breast and prostate, some of it was being used to suppress breast lactation in women who had just delivered babies, some of it was being used in agriculture, and some of it was being used—without FDA approval—as a morning-after pill.

In 1972 Belita Cowan was a health-care instructor at the University of Michigan's sprawling Ann Arbor campus. A dedicated consumer activist who now heads the National Women's Health Network, she started interviewing hundreds of women who had been given DES as a morning-after pill from 1968 on. Her interest was in learning how and when DES was being used, what precautions were taken regarding its use, and what follow-up there had been of students exposed to massive doses of the estrogens. She concluded her study in 1975 and that year presented her findings to the House Subcommittee on Health. She said—and her statement was never contradicted—that what was happening in Ann Arbor was indicative of what was happening elsewhere around the country:

- Some young women were being given the morning-after pill on two, three, and four different occasions, from which one can infer that they were using the morning-after pill as their principal means of contraception.

- Roughly half of the women were not asked for a personal medical history, to see if there was a history of cancer in the family. (Estrogens, including DES, have always been contraindicated for people with a history of cancer.)
- Roughly half of the women in her study were not given a pelvic or breast exam to judge their health.
- Only one out of four was followed up to see if DES actually worked in preventing pregnancy.
- Four out of five experienced nausea, and one out of three experienced vomiting.
- Three out of five said they would never take DES as a morning-after pill again. Although the reasons weren't stated in the survey, the high rate of nausea and increased consumer awareness apparently account for this.

At the time of Cowan's report, consumers and senators were under the mistaken impression that the FDA had approved DES for postcoital use two years earlier. The agency had sent out a bulletin to the nation's doctors telling them that DES was approved for certain limited uses: in the case of rape, incest, or other emergencies. The limitations were being imposed, agency officials later testified, because of the known potency of the drug. There was never any guideline as to what such "other emergencies" might be, but a compassionate doctor might see a distraught woman who said she had had unprotected intercourse and decide that her distress constituted an emergency.

Belita Cowan pointed out in her congressional testimony that women in critical need of postcoital contraception, especially those who had been victimized by rape or incest, would hardly be in a frame of mind to hear or understand the risks associated with estrogen use. Or the attending emergency-room physician might be insufficiently informed to explain the risks.

In fact, although the FDA bulletin had been sent—and had formed the basis for the use of the drug by physicians—official *approval* had never been given. This came out at the Senate hearings in 1975, conducted by Senator Edward M. Kennedy, when FDA Commissioner Alexander Schmidt announced that he would seek to have DES approved for postcoital use because he was concerned about its unauthorized use for this purpose. Such an approval by the FDA would not necessarily mean that its use for that purpose would increase, he said, but rather that the FDA would be better able to regulate its use.

Schmidt testified that the 1973 notice had actually been an an-

nouncement of what the FDA *intended* to do and not an announcement of the approval itself; the actual approval had never been given.
Kennedy called the 1973 notice "an inexcusable error" by the FDA.

It ought to be pointed out here that whether or not people thought
DES had been approved for postcoital use, no one was able to introduce any controlled, double-blind study showing that it actually works
as a morning-after pill. As Bruce Stadel, M.D., a federal health-care authority says, "Nine out of ten acts of intercourse don't result in conception anyway." If DES has a chance of working in only one out of ten
cases, why give it at all? Why douse the female body with a powerful
substance already associated with cancer?

Eli Lilly & Company made its own decision in 1974 that it would
not recommend DES for postcoital use, stating that it had neither conducted nor supported research showing DES was effective for this purpose. Lilly continued to make DES tablets, which it recommended for
other purposes, although any physician could certainly prescribe the
readily available Lilly tablets for use as a morning-after pill.

There is no known safe dosage tolerance for DES, no numerical level
at which one can say, "It is safe to have the body exposed to this
amount of DES, but unsafe for it to be exposed to any more." And
since there is no known safe level, and at least two million young
American women were exposed before birth to DES, what will happen
to them if they are then given DES as a morning-after pill? Consumer
advocates strongly urge DES-exposed women not to use estrogens or
DES. Other medical people say there is no indication that such an add-
on effect is harmful, but no one really knows.

Only one company ever filed an application with the FDA to market
the drug as a morning-after pill. In 1974 Tablicaps, Inc. of Franklin-
ville, New Jersey submitted to the FDA technical documents and promotional materials it intended to use. These were placed in the public
record of Senator Kennedy's health subcommittee. The president of
Tablicaps, Bela Jancsik, said in a recent telephone interview that the
company had never marketed the drug, since it didn't have FDA approval. However, excerpts from the papers Tablicaps filed with the
FDA are of value in showing how the commercial interests of profit-
making companies were once again brought to bear on DES.

In a proposed "Dear Mr. Buyer" letter DESMA (the company's
trademark name) would be marketed for "unprotected sexual exposure
... The need for such a product has been clearly established by studies
... which indicate that the market for a postcoital contraceptive will be

sizeable . . . DESMA (tm) will be heavily promoted and personal contacts by detailmen will be made to physicians, Planned Parenthood, and hospital clinics. It will be advertised in *ObGyn Journal, ObGyn News,* and *J.A.M.A."*

In another proposed marketing letter, one to be sent to pharmacists, drug wholesalers, and other business people whose commercial interests lie in influencing doctors, this statement appeared under the Tablicaps letterhead: "Desma is a postcoital contraceptive that may be used by every woman of childbearing age. As outlined by the Food and Drug Administration, Desma is for emergency use (in such situations as rape, incest, or where, in the physician's judgment, the patient's physical or mental well-being is in jeopardy) and should not be used as a routine method of contraception. Until now all that could be offered a female who did not want to be pregnant was an abortion—not very consoling for a woman in such a predicament." The statement then detailed the number of rapes reported annually, a number that might be significantly smaller than the total of reported and unreported rapes. It talked about rape crisis centers and the National Organization for Women's National Rape Task Force.

In another proposed marketing statement the company wrote: "Dear Doctor: TABLICAPS INC. introduced 'Desma,' the postcoital tablet, which will provide security in spontaneity . . . This mode of fertility control has received considerable attention as the optimum contraceptive since it does not compromise spontaneity of the sex act . . . Doctor, 'Desma' is for your patient who needs a highly effective, safe, birth control method the morning after." This sounds much like the earlier language and marketing philosophy behind the use of DES for pregnancy use: the safe drug that would be a convenience to patients, with no reference to potential side effects.

Roy Hertz, M.D., has headed the endocrinology branch of the National Cancer Institute, and formerly was the scientific director of the National Institute of Child Health and Human Development. In 1971 he testified at the same hearings at which Arthur L. Herbst and Peter Greenwald had testified about their findings of a rare vaginal cancer in DES daughters. Hertz testified on the subject of estrogens in general, with specific reference to DES: "Our inadequate knowledge concerning the relationship of estrogens to cancer in women is comparable with what was known about the association between lung cancer and cigarette smoking before extensive epidemiologic study delineated this overwhelmingly significant relationship." In effect, why use something that might be dangerous when the risk of danger is unknown?

15

DES ON THE DINNER TABLE

Each day during the cold spring of 1951 veteran Illinois mink rancher Henry J. Krueger walked out to his barns, waiting for his prize herd of 500 mink to deliver their litters. Mr. Krueger had been raising mink for twenty-five years. Each breeder in his herd had cost from $100 to $500, and each usually had a litter of 7 or 8 kittens.

But not that year.

"The whole herd was sterile, every last one of them. They all looked pregnant, big and fat, and they even had milk in them, like they were about to deliver. But nothing happened. I was nearly wiped out." Krueger had fed his mink herd the heads and necks of chickens raised with the new wonder drug DES, which was being used by poultry breeders to raise their chickens faster and more cheaply. The pellet of DES was implanted in the chickens' necks.

A number of fur-industry journals had published negative reports about the sterility DES-bred chickens apparently caused in breeding minks, but the word had never filtered down to the man from whom Mr. Krueger bought his chickens, who had been following the advice of the Department of Agriculture to raise chickens with DES.

"Don't matter what you did to 'em—froze the meat or chopped it up—that DES stayed in them. We ground the chicken heads up with other foods and fed it to the minks. I bought eighteen hundred pounds of chicken, at six cents a pound, and fed them with it. Some of the dogs and pigs got into the food, and they went sterile too."

Mr. Krueger took three of the sterile mink to be autopsied at the University of Wisconsin's animal science lab. As might have been predicted by the pioneering work of Dodds, Parkes, and Noble in 1938, the autopsies showed that DES had somehow kept the mink from getting pregnant. Since the female minks had been mated, their bodies thought that a pregnancy was taking place, and so the animals went through what was in effect a false pregnancy. "They looked pregnant," the eighty-four-year-old rancher said when I talked to him. "But it was all fat."

Normally 15 percent of the herd would be expected to be sterile. But with the new miracle drug DES, virtually 100 percent of the herd was sterile. He got only 3 mink kittens instead of 3,500. "Since they were meant to be breeders, and were sterile, I had to do away with the whole herd," Mr. Krueger said.

At least five other established midwestern mink ranchers that year came close to financial ruin because their breeder minks turned out to be sterile after being fed DES-dosed chickens. Their congressman filed a special-interest bill on their behalf, seeking a special appropriation of $268,185.30 for all of them, to compensate them for their losses. The bill passed the House and Senate and was signed by the President, but neither Mr. Krueger nor any of the others saw a dime of it.

"I can't tell you how many times we were in the courthouse, fighting with the government. The Department of Agriculture stopped it. They said 'if we paid you, we'll have to pay everyone who's lost animals.' " A government analysis at the time stated that the Department of Agriculture "knew or should have known" that the chicken wastes, tainted with DES, would sterilize the animals.

A federal official recently told me he was unaware of the incident.

During the legal wrangling, Mr. Krueger said, agents from the Federal Bureau of Investigation came out to his ranch to review his books. "They said there was a difference of one mink pelt between what I was claiming and what they could find. They went over my books for days."

Mr. Krueger borrowed money, made other arrangements, and renewed his herd of five hundred breeding mink. He retired twenty years ago. "But I'll tell you, I've been worried about it ever since, what that stuff does to you."

Henry J. Krueger is symbolic of America's rude awakening to the power of diethylstilbestrol used in animals, a widespread and dangerous use that the country nearly ignored, lulled by industry and livestock officials who saw the drug as a cheap way to raise animals faster and more economically.

DES was a known cancer-causing agent, and yet it was legally used in this country for decades to stimulate growth in chicken, beef cattle, and sheep, animals that would later end up on the nation's dinner tables. It was used despite the fact that no one could conclusively say that residues of it did not remain in the T-bone steaks and chicken breasts and lamb chops eaten by unsuspecting consumers for thirty years. Its use by powerful corporations and influential feedlot owners was, one way or the other, protected by the Food and Drug Administration, which was excoriated in 1973 by a congressional committee for inadequate supervision, illegal actions, indecision, delaying tactics, and contradictory actions regarding DES.

One federal official (who has spent years tracking down DES use in agriculture) said: "Industry has a pathological fear that new tests showing the toxicity of other big money makers will be developed, just like tests for DES were developed. The closest thing to evil I have ever encountered was the continued use of this stuff despite all the knowledge about its harm to people."

Other nations have not waited for America's response before banning DES, and DES-raised meat, from their shores. All of the Common Market nations did it by the 1960s; Italy refused to accept Danish ham; Canada refused to buy U.S. meat; along the winding streets of the chic Seventh Arrondissement in Paris or out in the small village centers, the butcher shops, or *charcuteries*, put up signs saying *"Non hormones."*

Drugs have been used for generations to treat sick animals, including animals later slaughtered for food. The common wisdom was that as long as the medication was for the prevention or cure of a specific illness and given for only a short period of time, there would be no danger to consumers. By World War II, however, the science of veterinary medicine had progressed rapidly, following the same pharmaceutical path as human medicine. Livestock breeders were able not only to cure diseases but, by using medicated foods and chemical implants, able also to control the rate and speed at which the animals developed—turning the pasture into a sort of outdoor laboratory. By 1971 the use of medications in the nation's livestock industry had gotten so complex that a congressional committee concluded that 80 percent of all meat, chicken, and eggs produced in America came from medicated animals. One of the most popular medications was DES.

Hormones regulate the balance and amount of lean and fat in body tissue and the conversion of food into tissue. Very soon after the 1938 synthesis of DES, it was realized that this female sex hormone could be easily used to manipulate the growth of animals. For generations farmers had fattened poultry up by castrating the males, which eliminated the production of male sex hormones associated with harder, leaner bodies. One early use of DES was as a chemical castrator: as a female sex hormone, it suppressed the production of male hormones and added feminizing qualities to the animal's chemical system.

The same qualities that made DES attractive for pregnancy use—low cost and the convenience of taking it by mouth—soon contributed to glowing reports of its use in animals: low cost and its pellet form, the animal equivalent of the pill.

Sir Charles Dodds wrote throughout his career about the use of DES as a growth stimulant in animals and stated that such a use was safe if it was discontinued one week before the animal was slaughtered for market. The pellets of DES were implanted in the necks of cattle, chickens, and sheep. Dodds reported that it had the effect of making old cock birds saleable as poultry; after several months of life with DES pellets embedded in the neck, they had increased in weight, mainly through the addition of fat on the bones, and had a more pleasing, juicier taste. But as a precaution Dodds late in life warned his daughter-in-law, Lady Marian Dodds, "never to use the gizzard in with the giblets."

In this country the FDA received the first application to use DES in poultry in 1945, a request that was granted in 1947. DES had always been known to be a cancer-causing agent, but at the time, and for years later, there were no tests to show that traces of DES remained in the chickens after slaughter. Some poultry growers removed the pellet a day or two before slaughter. (Later, more sophisticated tests showed that traces remained even if the pellet were removed as much as two weeks before slaughter.)

Recent research, however, has shown that minute traces of DES do remain in the slaughtered animal and pass on to the human consumer. Such a development would not have surprised Dodds, however, who told his son that "in the 50 years he had been in science there had been more developments than in the last 400 years," and he didn't know what the future would bring.

In 1954 the addition of DES to the feed of beef cattle was approved, and the next year pellets were allowed to be implanted in cattle. In 1957 the use of DES in lambs was added to the approved list. Fairly soon 300 million cattle per year (or 75 percent of American cattle slaughtered for table use) had been raised on DES. That means that three out of every four hamburger patties, sirloin steaks, T-bone steaks, rib roasts, flank steaks, and every other conceivable cut from the corner butcher had come from an animal with DES in its system. In addition, it was estimated that each week in this country 55,000 calves, 1.29 million pigs, 277,000 lambs, and 540,000 cattle were slaughtered with DES residue in them. The same percentages are believed to be true for chickens.

At the same time, during the 1950s, there was a growing awareness of the impact that the environment has on human health. The air we breathe, the water we drink, and the food we eat were all believed to have an influence on human health, or the lack of it. There was a growing opinion in the medical community that environmental factors—factors that exist in the workplace, or the marketplace, in the home, or in substances put into the body—might have some relationship to the development of cancer.

One result of this was the development in 1957 of a new method of testing to discover whether DES residues remained in chickens after slaughter. They did—up to twenty or thirty parts per billion in the skin fat of treated poultry. But legislators were powerless to regulate the livestock and chemical industries. In September 1958, in an attempt to correct this imbalance of power, Congress passed the Food Additives Amendment to the Food, Drug, and Cosmetic Act of 1938, regulating the substances that can legally be added to food. The regulation included the famous Delaney Amendment, which banned all foods with any traces of cancer-causing agents from the marketplace. The next year the Department of Health, Education, and Welfare decided that DES belonged in this category, and Secretary Arthur S. Flemming requested DES makers to stop using or selling the product for poultry.

Industry strongly objected. Ban DES in poultry and soon you'll be banning it in cattle. The poultry industry went to court. For the next seven years, until a federal appeals court in 1966 upheld the ban in a case known as *Bell* v. *Goddard*, most poultry in this country was sold with DES traces in its fatty tissue.

The Delaney Amendment was controversial in its absolutist approach. The result of years of thought and investigation by Representative James Delaney of New York, its forty-seven words rocked the chemical, pharmaceutical, and manufacturing industires. The original amendment read: "No additive shall be deemed to be safe if it is found to induce cancer when ingested by man or animal, or if it is found after tests which are appropriate for the evaluation of the safety of food additives to induce cancer in man or animal." No exceptions were allowed, and that is what disturbed advocates of popular industrial and agricultural chemicals: there were no loopholes.

The language and intent of the Delaney amendment were neither frivolous nor casual. Delaney, a veteran congressman, had headed the Select Committee to Investigate the Use of Chemicals in Food ever since the committee was formed in 1949. It had been created in the wake of the widespread increase in the use of chemicals in the growing of raw agricultural products, as well as in processing foods for flavor, preservation, and packaging. The Delaney committee held hearings throughout much of the 1950s, and the testimony had a major bearing on the ability of Congressman Delaney to get his amendment passed in 1958.

There were also hearings on Capitol Hill regarding substances that could be added to food as coloring agents, which were often used simply to make food products look more appealing to consumers. As initially proposed, such color additives would also be banned if they were found to be carcinogenic. In 1960 there were more hearings; one witness was Thomas Carney, Ph.D., a Lilly vice-president and also chairman of the Committee for the Study of Carcinogenic Substances of the Pharmaceutical Manufacturers Association.

During his testimony Carney said: "[Diethylstilbestrol's] safety in man and animals has been fully established for years . . . Under the Delaney amendment, this completely safe and very valuable chemical could never have been developed and introduced in animal feeds and its many benefits to farmers and consumers would never have been realized . . . I should emphasize that there is no detectable residue in beef or sheep which have been fed stilbestrol under recommended conditions; so it cannot cause any side effects . . ."

Science is at the mercy of its tools; a substance can't be measured if the measuring stick doesn't exist. In 1960 the best yardstick for measuring DES only went down to ten parts per billion, which by scientific standards today is considered grossly inadequate. When that measuring tool was applied to chickens, DES was found in the fatty tissues. Not for another eleven years was that yardstick improved, and when it was calibrated down to two parts per billion, DES residues were found in cattle. Two parts per billion is the equivalent to 1.5 drops in a 25,000-gallon tank.

It has always been FDA policy to insist that the manufacturer of an animal drug has the sole responsibility for developing practical methods of testing whether residues of the drug exist in animal tissues after slaughter. The FDA is by statute responsible only for validating those tests. But for years the FDA permitted manufacturers to market DES without developing such tests. At one point, according to congressional documents, the government had to pay $48,250 in taxpayers' money to a private research organization to develop the tests that were rightfully the responsibility of the industries.

Thomas Carney told the House committee that DES was also widely used in medicine and that "the average therapeutic dose in human beings is probably closer to 0.5 to 1.0 milligram per day." That may have been the average dose of all DES tablets taken for all purposes, but the standard Lilly dosage schedule recommended for pregnancy started at 5 milligrams and went up to 125 milligrams each day, according to Lilly's own product brochures. However, testimony of people such as Carney and the absence of any conclusive connection between DES use in animals and harm in people apparently reassured many congressmen.

The Delaney Amendment was modified in 1962 to permit the use of substances that are known to be cancer-causing as long as their residue don't show up in the feed chain. The section, informally known as the DES clause, in effect permits undetected residues to exist in the food chain. Such residues would be detected if tests were run that searched for them, with instruments sensitive enough to find them. But the instruments didn't exist, and the testing wasn't done, or wasn't done very extensively or with much enthusiasm, for more than a decade, until the Boston studies came out in 1971 showing the association between vaginal cancer in young girls and those mothers who had taken DES during pregnancy.

In *Sowing the Wind,* author Harrison Wellford recounts that Assistant Secretary of Agriculture Richard Lyng, a former top executive for the meat-packing lobby, announced after the 1971 cancer scare that "no red meat containing detectable levels of DES has reached the consumer." Wellford points out that Lyng based his information on 1970 FDA tests done on only 192 steers, a small number out of the more than 31 million slaughtered under federal inspection; and the testing had been done with instruments that could detect residues only down to ten parts per billion.

In fact, in 1970 the FDA doubled the allowable dosage of DES that could be given to animals, from a maximum of 10 milligrams in feed to a new high of 20 milligrams, despite the absence of a reliable test to determine how much DES was ending up on the dinner table. And in doing so the FDA blatantly ignored a 1970 report issued by an advisory group within the office of the U.S. Surgeon General, which stated that even low levels of toxic substances should be considered unsafe, especially if there was no test available for determining safety. "The principle of a zero tolerance for carcinogenic exposures should be retained in all areas of legislation." Because some FDA scientists disagreed with the report, the warning was ignored.

Whatever standards were in effect, however, when it comes down to reality, we should realize that we're talking about small businessmen whose inventory is on four legs, whose motto is "get the job done," and whose work day lasts long past sundown. If they disagreed with the requirement to stop giving DES to animals a few hours or days before slaughter, would they still abide by the requirement? And would anyone on a feedlot, including federal inspectors, discover any such omissions, using instruments considered even at the time to be insensitive to minute amounts of DES? Would a rancher clean out the feed buckets thoroughly if he mixed DES with the feed (as opposed to implanting it behind the ear)? Would he use DES to prevent miscarriages in cows, just as it was used to prevent miscarriages in women? An FDA spokesman told me that DES had never been approved for use in preventing miscarriages in animals. But Opal Cannon of Albany, Georgia, remembers coming home from her doctor and telling her rancher husband that she had just received a prescription for DES to help her carry their baby. "Why, that's the same stuff I use for my cows, to keep 'em from miscarrying," her husband exclaimed.

The DES subject faded on Capitol Hill in the years following the 1962 passage of the Delaney Amendment, until the *New England Journal of Medicine* published the Herbst, Ulfelder, Poskanzer article showing the association between young women with clear-cell adenocarcinoma and DES use by their mothers during pregnancy. Then Representative L. H. Fountain, from North Carolina, chaired hearings of his Subcommittee on Government Operations regarding DES. He covered all the fields touched by the drug—its uses in pregnancy, as a morning-after pill, and in livestock and agriculture.

Cancer was a constant topic of conversation at the hearings, held in Room 2154 of the Rayburn House Office Building. Special attention was given to the question of whether cancer could be stimulated by the minute amounts of DES found in meat. One theory claims that cancer is caused on a molecule-by-molecule basis. On November 11, 1971, there was this revealing conversational byplay between congressional consultant Gilbert S. Goldhammer and witness Mortimer B. Lipsett, M.D., associate scientific director of reproductive biology at the National Institute of Child Health and Human Development. The discussion began with Goldhammer and Lipsett acknowledging that existing testing methods could detect DES residues down to only two parts per billion. But what if there were residues at one part per billion?

Goldhammer said: "For a residue of one part per billion, if we consume 145 grams, or five ounces [of liver], we would have ingested 340 trillion molecules of DES. . . . Do you perceive in that situation the complete absence of any hazard?" Lipsett answered, "No, sir . . . in terms of potential hazard one would have to say yes [there is a potential hazard]."

Roy Hertz, M.D., former chief of the endocrinology branch of the National Cancer Institute and one of the nation's leading cancer researchers, testified that cancer in human beings takes ten to twenty years to develop, and that the Herbst study had borne this out—the young women in his study had developed cancer ten to twenty years after exposure to DES, a known carcinogen. Congressman Fountain pointed out that other witnesses had testified that DES tended to concentrate in the liver of cattle treated with it, and that beef liver was used in some prepared baby foods. Did Hertz have an opinion on that, even if the amount was as low as two parts per billion?

"I would say the hazard of any amount in any foods to be ingested by human subjects, and, for that matter, pets around the house, would constitute a substantial hazard which we would be much better off without . . . I would strongly recommend the elimination of the hazard of this material entering the human food supply irrespective of the economic cost involved." The only conceivable reason to justify the use of DES, Hertz stated, was in a "famine."

Fountain asked FDA Commissioner Charles C. Edwards, M.D.: "[Can] you or your staff unequivocally assure the American people at this time that no one need fear the effect of minute quantities of DES in animal tissue?"

After some technical discussions Edwards replied, "I think we all agree that we can provide reasonable assurance that this will not happen." He said that the current detection methods that showed DES residues in meat down to two parts per billion were, in effect, showing that 99.5 percent of all DES had been eliminated from the meat.

Fountain said: "It sounds good on its face, but when you analyze it, I am not so sure . . . I do not know whether anybody has or has not developed cancer from DES residues in meat. I do not believe anyone really knows. But what I do know is that cancer mortality rates are on the increase and we do not know why. We do not know how these carcinogens act on the body cells to render them cancerous. That is precisely why Congress enacted the Delaney clause—to protect the public in the absence of such knowledge."

When the testing was finally and effectively conducted, spurred on by this angry congressman, DES traces *were* found in cattle and sheep livers—sometimes at comparatively high levels of 15 and 37 parts per billion respectively.

Manufacturers of DES for use in animal feeds included dozens of small firms around the country, as well as the Hess & Clark division of Rhone-Poulenc, Inc., and Vineland Laboratories, which later fought an FDA ban in court and eventually lost. One of the biggest producers was the Elanco Products division of Eli Lilly & Company. Fundamentally the same formula was used for making the DES given to livestock and that taken by people.

Elanco had a licensing arrangement with Iowa State University in Ames, Iowa, and the university produced some of the most favorable analyses of DES use in livestock, *Washington Post* reporter Morton Mintz wrote in 1972. In his book *The Politics of Cancer* Samuel S. Epstein, M.D., quoted a report of the Agribusiness Accountability Project showing that ISU had received a royalty of $2.9 million and that Lilly had sales of the product of more than $58 million.

Economic concerns, as suggested at a 1971 congressional hearing, were of constant importance in the battle to keep DES in use. The livestock industry has always maintained that animals could be raised about 10 percent faster and with approximately 10–13 percent less feed *with* DES than without it. A government report late in 1971, endorsed by the meat industry, said that banning DES from use in livestock production would raise the cost of meat 3½ cents a pound, or $3.85 a year per person, based on average consumption. Not insignificantly, banning DES would also cost American meat producers at least $460 million annually in extra expenses.

The remarkable thing about the insistence of feedlot owners and manufacturers on using DES is that, even if one overlooks the fact that DES is carcinogenic in people, it clearly isn't any healthier for animals.

Sir Charles Dodds had pointed out that the old cock birds treated with DES did gain weight, but it was extra fat. Some American ranchers and meat buyers complained to their congressmen in the late 1950s that DES-raised meat had more fat in solid masses on the tissue and less marbling (wisps of fat) in the lean meat, and therefore was harder to sell in the open market. There were also anecdotal reports about a personality dysfunction in DES cattle, which had caused some steers to die as a result. Ranchers call it "bulling and riding," but Charles Dodds had used a more clinical term: nymphomania. Steers implanted with DES become feminized; if too much DES is used, an artificial "heat" is produced. Other cattle will try to "bull," or "ride," the DES steer, and often serious abrasions will occur. One government report showed that 7 percent of all "buller" steers had died from this. The abrasions occurred in part because of weakened pelvic ligaments, as Dodds and others had noted. Ranchers know that all cattle tend toward this behavior but observed that DES steers seemed to be more prone to it.

Despite these curious effects on animals, anything that could help get herds of cattle out of the feedlot and into the packing houses faster and at less cost was desirable—at least to the makers and suppliers of the chemical. Estimates at the time were that a 1,000-pound steer raised on DES feed or implanted with a DES pellet behind his floppy ear could be readied for slaughter one month sooner than an untreated animal, saving the feedlot owner about 500 pounds of feed. In an era of increasing grain and other prices, that represented a considerable saving.

And those numbers also had a political implication, according to testimony on Capitol Hill. Meat prices were already rising drastically as a result of increased fuel costs (the result of increases by the Arab oil-producing cartel) and increased feed costs (the result of the sale of American grain to the Soviet Union). Politicians feared the voters' wrath at the ballot box if they voted to ban DES and, by implication, contributed to the rising cost of meat.

FDA Commissioner Edwards testified in 1971 that cattlemen would be required to withdraw DES from beef at least seven days before slaughter, as opposed to the two-days-before-slaughter standard that had previously existed. In mid-July of 1972 the FDA announced that DES would be banned as a feed additive, although existing stocks of DES-treated feed could stay on the market until 1973. Interestingly, that ban did *not* apply to the equally popular method of using DES, implanting a pellet behind an animal's ear.

On August 15, 1972, Senator Edward M. Kennedy, testifying before Representative Fountain's committee, stated that the 1971 FDA changes had been brought about only after a lawsuit had been filed by the National Resources Defense Council. Even with the new regula-

tions, Kennedy testified, there were fifty-eight incidents of DES violations, with only one brought to trial. Kennedy had held his own hearings into DES, and he concluded that the FDA "has effectively abdi-
cated its responsibility in this area ... DES is dangerous for the
American people."

After hearings are held in Washington it is customary for a lengthy
report to be prepared for the Congress, summarizing the testimony and
drawing conclusions. On December 10, 1973, the report by Representative Fountain's Intergovernmental Relations Subcommittee was completed. It presented a scathing picture of the Food and Drug Administration, charged by statute with protecting the nation's health. Among
its findings were these:

> FDA regulation of diethylstilbestrol (DES) for use as a drug in animal
> feed was inadequate because of errors in judgment and deficiencies in
> administration. . . . There was little or no monitoring of the meat supply
> for the detection of DES residues until 1967. . . . FDA's failure to re-
> quire submission of a practicable test method for DES residues resulted
> in the needless and unwarranted expenditure of public funds to develop
> and validate such a method. . . . FDA misjudged the capacity of the
> DES in feed to cross-contaminate nonmedicated foods. . . . FDA regula-
> tion of DES in animal feeds was marked by indecision and contradictory
> actions. Its June 1972 proposal to ban DES was only a tactic to delay
> decisive regulatory action. . . . FDA acted illegally in permitting ship-
> ment and use of DES for five months after the August 4, 1972 DES ban
> went into effect.

The report contained other extraordinary attacks on the FDA: "FDA
erroneously claimed that. . . . Congress intended to weaken the Delaney
anticancer clause. . . . FDA was tardy in warning physicians that the use
of DES during pregnancy is unsafe. . . . FDA made regulatory decisions
concerning DES use in pregnancy on the basis of alleged analyses for
which no records exist. [FDA officials had told a Congressional committee they were reviewing the Herbst and Greenwald cancer data before taking action on their findings but later could not produce a single
piece of paper to back up their statements that they actually did such a
review]. . . . FDA has excessively delayed regulatory decisions concerning some widely used animal feed drugs of questionable safety." Among
other things, the report recommended that "FDA take the necessary
steps to insure that the Delaney anticancer clause as amended in 1962
will be strictly enforced so that the public will not be exposed to detectable residues of carcinogenic drugs."

Once goaded, the FDA did in fact step up its pace of regulatory activity. In 1973 it banned DES from animal feed, a ban that was overturned by a court in 1974. The FDA tried again in 1976, and industry fought the ban again; in 1979 the FDA also banned the use of implants in cattle. After the 1979 ban, however, there were widespread violations by more than 300 ranchers and feedlots, according to published FDA figures. The courts upheld the ban on November 24, 1980, and the FDA seized 170,000 pounds of meat, liver, and kidney from a Kansas feedlot owner. The government lost the Kansas case when a federal judge ruled on May 7, 1981, that DES in meat would not harm people and therefore the meat should not be held. At the moment, however, DES is legally forbidden to be used in animals.

During all this time as the FDA wobbled, the Congress shouted, and the courts reviewed, manufacturers of DES were in effect placing the responsibility on consumers to protect themselves against a hazard, even though the manufacturers themselves did not have the measuring tools to prove that the drug presented no danger.

Does this all matter? Are lawyers, legislators, and journalists arguing a mere technicality, scaring the public without reason? A number of anecdotes argue otherwise.

Duane E. Townsend, M.D., is a Los Angeles gynecologist and a member of the federal DES Task Force. In one interview with me, he said that he had once treated two young women with the classic signs of DES daughters: adenosis and the cockscomb cervix. Their mothers denied "taking anything" during pregnancy. "Finally I asked about chicken necks. The mother said they did eat a lot of chicken necks." This is certainly a rare occurrence, but we are talking about a known cancer-causing agent, a drug of unusual strength and power. Townsend is a conservative physician, one not given to medical hyperbole. "The scary thing about DES," he said, "is, who knows?"

William C. Hobson is director of the Primate Research Institute at New Mexico State University. His interest is in learning the impact that hormones will have on rhesus monkeys—the primate species most similar to humans. In a paper published in 1982 in England, Hobson and colleagues G. B. Fuller, D. E. Yates, and E. D. Helton reported that their studies "demonstrated unequivocally that exposure of rhesus monkeys to DES either *in utero* or during the first year of life causes profound changes in postnatal endocrine function. Thus, the rhesus infant could serve as a model for predicting the long-term reproductive effects of *in utero* or postnatal exposure to hormonally active drugs and environmental agents."

What does this mean? At the very least, DES has an impact on the way the body responds and will respond throughout life. Just as psychologists June Machover Reinisch and Melissa Hines have shown that DES has an impact on the way human responsibility can be influenced by DES, Hobson and colleagues have taken a look at the way it influences the body's chemistry. Their study shows that DES given to monkeys *in utero* or just after birth influences the rate and levels of two major sex hormones—follicle-stimulating hormone (FSH) and luteinizing hormone (LH). These hormones are widely understood to control the rate and development of sexual maturity in people. DES changes the rate and time at which these hormones interact in monkeys. It might do the same in people.

In monkeys DES changes the chemical patterns, both at the moment of exposure and for years afterward. The paper by Hobson and his collagueus added: "It is evident that the transition [of the chemical agents from one state to another before puberty] can be functionally modified during fetal development [by outside chemical forces]. Although the mechanism and the site of action of DES is unknown, the potential of the DES-treated fetus and infant rhesus model for studying the mechanism of sexual differentiation is immense. DES has proven in this study to be a useful endocrine probe that can be used to investigate the control mechanisms that govern primate sexual differentiation and postnatal sexual development."

In one way or another—either in chicken, beef, or lamb—DES has been legally in the food chain and on the dinner table for most of the years between 1947 and 1980. During all that time its potency was known, its potential side effects were known, the difficulty in detecting it was known—and these facts were ignored by businessmen making money and by some bureaucrats whose own colleagues later berated them for timid, contradictory, and sometimes illegal actions regarding DES. The industry officials who lobbied for DES were lobbying in their own self-interest and never for the consumer. Can a saving of $3.85 a year on the price of meat really be worth the adenosis and cockscomb cervix in the two young women examined by Duane Townsend?

You didn't have to be pregnant to get DES in America: you just had to have a good meal.

16

DES CONSUMERS' MOVEMENT

With the publication of the Herbst, Ulfelder, Poskanzer article in the spring of 1971, women all across the country found themselves reading about DES in newspapers and magazines, hearing about it on radio and television news shows, getting calls from friends and relatives—wasn't *that* the drug they'd taken?

DES mother Fran Fishbane read about the Herbst report in *The New York Times* delivered to the front door of her Plainview, Long Island, home; Pat Cody, a DES mother, remembers the exact day—April 23, 1971—she read about the Herbst report in the San Francisco *Chronicle* delivered to her Berkeley, California, house; Andrea Goldstein's mother called her in Boston and told her; Mary Patton's gynecologist, George Speck, M.D., advised her about it during a routine visit in his Alexandria, Virginia, office; Dave McWaters, in San Francisco, remembers his mother telling him that when she read about the report she felt relieved because "DES doesn't affect men."

In 1971 there wasn't much to be done: if a mother knew her daughter was DES-exposed, she could tell her or arrange for a gynecological examination to check for cancer. None of the other reproductive tract problems in women or men was known for nearly another decade. But there was a great deal to be *felt*. "So many women felt so alone," Fran Fishbane remembers. "I felt an anxiety I had never felt before in my life. I thought I had it all—college degrees, a good marriage, children—and then this. I know the hurt of watching girls that age— they're just children. I thought, if there was some way I could get people to stop saying, 'I thought I was alone in this.' "

The wife of an attorney/businessman, Fran Fishbane has an advanced degree in psychology and is a painter whose work decorates her split-level home. In a story that is the parallel of efforts of people in a wide variety of fields who found themselves feeling frustrated and alone when seeking help for problems they never anticipated and didn't cause—such as mental retardation, Toxic Shock, chemical waste sites such as Love Canal—she started spreading the word to women in her suburban community that there was a health problem they ought to know about.

"I put a notice in *The Pennysaver*, a small weekly advertising throwaway paper distributed in our area. I said we would have a meeting to talk about it. A lot of people showed up, mainly women. There were very few men." They consulted together: who were the doctors to go to, what should be looked for, why couldn't they see their own records, what did certain phrases mean, should a girl who hadn't started to menstruate have a gynecological exam?

"I made myself familiar with every medical report—I believed we should read every one that came out. I made myself familiar with everything about a woman from the waist down. I got medical dictionaries, I went to libraries, I talked to specialists. I wanted to know as much as the doctors did, and I think I did."

Like other women trying to compete against established interests, she didn't have plush offices to work in. She pushed aside some chairs, made some extra shelf space, and set to work in the basement of her house. Later she got office space at Long Island Jewish Hospital. "I had never heard of a grass-roots movement before," she said when asked what it was like to start one.

At the same time, around the country, other women were doing the same thing. Small, informal groups were set up in Rockville (Maryland), Boston, Portland (Oregon), Philadelphia, Santa Monica, and San Francisco. Sometimes the women worked out of their homes; sometimes they were given desk space in the offices of newly emerging women's groups. Their members often talked with members of other single-issue groups (such as those concerned with air pollution, noise pollution, or violence on television) to gather information on tactics and strategy. And by working with established consumer groups—such as the Coalition for the Medical Rights of Women in San Francisco, or chapters of the National Organization for Women, or community health groups, or health-care clinics—they became part of the larger network of interested consumers. The phrase "networking" became a part of the contemporary vocabulary, particularly with reference to women's issues, to indicate small local groups that had informal affiliations with larger, national ones.

Always these DES people worked long hours, with no pay, trying to get local TV stations, radio talk shows, and newspaper reporters to listen to their stories, to help them get the word out. Fran Fishbane worked downstairs in her Long Island home; Phyllis Wetherill worked in the basement of her white brick Washington, D.C., house, where her typewriter sat in front of her children's books; Pat Cody used a desk at the Coalition for the Medical Rights of Women, in San Francisco, and spread the word at Cody's Books (in Berkeley), an important center of social and cultural events which she and her husband had founded.

At first the interested people were mainly DES mothers concerned about their daughters. Gradually husbands came into the fold, then DES sons joined DES daughters. Their aim was to gather information and also to alert every woman who had taken any drug during the three decades of the 1940s, fifties, and sixties to find out if the drug had been DES. But sometimes people were as desperate for someone to talk to as for practical advice.

"At the DES office once we had three people call up in a short period of time and say they were suicidal," Fran Fishbane remembers. "They were desperate. Once a man called up from Philadelphia. He said he was too ashamed to go to a doctor. At erection his penis was only an inch and a half long. He started to cry. Another time a woman called up from Seattle. She had cancer, she was threatening suicide. I kept her talking on the phone while I told a doctor near me. He called a friend of his in Seattle, who called the police. I was still on the phone with her when they broke her door down. I heard everything, the sound of the pills she was going to use, the sound of the door crashing open. The girl later had a hysterectomy, and then she got married."

During federal hearings in the 1970s on DES use as a growth stimulant in animals, and then—after it had been banned for use during pregnancy—on its use as a morning-after contraceptive pill, Fishbane and other women lobbied their congressmen and knocked on doors, drumming up support for their position that a dangerous chemical was being foisted on the public despite knowledge about its risks. But now this public could no longer be described as "unknowing"; they *knew* about DES, and they wanted others to know as well.

"I believe in our society companies are in business to make money. The bottom line is economics," Fran said. But, she felt, no longer could they make money with a product she and others felt was dangerous.

In 1974, in response to congressional and consumer-group pressure, the National Cancer Institute funded the DES/Adenosis project. The DESAD project was designed to gather all known risks and facts about DES exposure. Fran Fishbane was asked to be a member of the group representing consumers. So was Phyllis Wetherill, and Andrea Goldstein testified before the group as a DES daughter.

Fishbane began lobbying her state representatives in Albany for passage of a bill that would set up screening clinics for DES-exposed people and launch a publicity campaign to urge people to find out if they were exposed. In order to convince one key state representative to support her she devised a unique strategy. The legislator was a die-hard right-to-lifer, opposed to all abortions, and she convinced him that the medical complications of DES destroyed a woman's body the same way an abortion in his view destroyed an unborn life. "When I talked to him I connected right-to-life with DES. I said, 'We need our bodies.' " The legislator lent his support.

In 1977 members of local groups concerned with DES met in New York City to discuss forming a national group. In 1978 they received a grant from the Ms. Foundation, set up by sponsors of *Ms.* magazine, and held a conference in Washington, D.C. They chose the name "DES Action, National" to indicate that there was a national organization and also to show that active units existed on the state and local levels as well. Fran Fishbane was elected the group's first president. There were originally seven chapters; today there are more than two dozen, with new ones forming every month, according to current president Nancy Adess.

Phyllis Wetherill later split from DES Action to form her own information service, DES Registry, which concentrates on providing detailed statistical analyses of the various medical studies on DES-exposed people. (A complete list of names and addresses of consumer organizations appears in the Appendix.)

The goal of DES Action, National was to identify all DES-exposed people, to provide referral and follow-up care, to develop networks of information, and to offer a forum (a newsletter) through which members could keep up with the latest medical and legal information and exchange common views and experiences. The group also wanted to act as a counterforce to what it felt was the all-too-frequent refusal of doctors to tell patients whether or not they were DES-exposed, and their outright denial or lies to women in the face of specific knowledge. The group also hoped to counteract the hesitancy of legislators or health officials to do anything about the DES problem.

As was common during the days of an expanding federal role in consumer issues, many of the ideas and concerns of women such as Fran Fishbane and Phyllis Wetherill were embodied in federal actions and programs. HEW Secretary Joseph Califano issued a health advisory to the nation's four hundred thousand doctors, informing them of the risk of DES exposure and requesting that they search their records for the names of women who might have received DES prescriptions in years past. Other government agencies issued medical brochures (aimed at doctors) and easy-to-understand pamphlets (for consumers) explaining what DES was, why women might have taken it, and what they and their children should do now.

In 1978 New York became the first state to pass DES-related legislation. Fran Fishbane (head of both DES Action, National and her state DES group) was present when Governor Hugh Carey signed the bill. One newspaper story at the time credited her with chief responsibility for the legislation, which established screening clinics throughout the state, a voluntary registry of DES people, educational programs for doctors and nurses, and made it illegal in New York State for an insurance company to deny coverage to anyone because of DES exposure. Other states, including Maryland and California, have passed similar legislation. At the signing ceremony Carey said that his late wife, Helen, had taken DES in two of her pregnancies and had died from breast cancer, which some medical professionals say could be related to DES exposure.

The years, however, have been hard for Fran Fishbane. In part because of her day-and-night efforts in the DES consumer field, her own health has been weakened. Physical movement for her is painful and conversations are often difficult. Several years ago, she said, she was in a hospital recovering from an illness. A doctor "rushed in and started yelling at me, saying I'd mentioned his name on television as someone who'd prescribed DES. I had been on television, but I hadn't used his name. I was too sick then to respond or even call the nurse." Then she added, speaking of the incident but addressing the whole DES experience, "Who ever thinks of a thing like that happening when it's not your fault?"

Sidney M. Wolfe, M.D., is the kind of doctor who drives most other doctors nuts. He is a doctor who does not hesitate to criticize other doctors, and he never hesitates to speak out when he thinks physicians—or others—are wrong. As head of the Ralph Nader-founded Public Citizen's Health Research Group, he performs on a wide-ranging basis the same type of consumer-oriented watchdog functions that Fran Fishbane performs on an *ad hoc*, single-issue basis. He is a part of the movement that strives to keep an influential consumer-interest force in Washington to match the powerful lobbies representing manufacturers and business interests which have so often successfully kept DES and other products like it on the medical shelf. "DES is an excellent example of how drug companies behave," he said in an interview, "how they take advantage of the ways doctors act, and how they make millions of dollars by ignoring evidence of a drug's harmfulness, by failing to get evidence that it is effective, and then by marketing a product that plays on fears and misconceptions."

In 1972 Wolfe learned of Belita Cowan's University of Michigan study on the misuse of DES as a morning-after pill. He fired off a letter to the school in an attempt to get the policy changed. At the same time, Public Citizen, a Nader organization, was compiling massive documentation on the use of DES as an animal growth stimulant, much of which was later used in congressional hearings.

Wolfe confronted the DES issue again in late 1977 when the Public Citizen's Litigation Group (another Nader affiliate, with which Wolfe was working) used the federal Freedom of Information Act to obtain the unreleased data that showed, Wolfe claimed, that DES mothers had a "significant increase in breast cancer and other hormone-related cancer." Medical people from the University of Chicago denied his interpretation. Wolfe has not backed away from his conclusions.

Wolfe put his conclusions in a December 12, 1977, letter to HEW Secretary Joseph Califano. He called for "long overdue" federal actions banning DES and other estrogens for use as morning-after pills and in the food supply of animals. In 1978, Califano created the DES task force, with Wolfe as one of its outside consultants. (Others were Fran Fishbane, Phyllis Wetherill, Arthur Herbst, Howard Ulfelder, and author Barbara Seaman.) The task force was only the third ever created by HEW, a reflection in part of the considerable weight industrial figures normally swing in government circles. (The other two had been the HEW task force on tobacco, and one on asbestos.)

The stated purpose of the DES task force was to bring together in a comprehensive fashion everything that was known about DES and present it in a logical, readable, and reassuring fashion. The popular perception of the drug then mainly concerned cancer; the reproductive and other risks later associated with it were largely unknown. At the time, it was estimated that 4 DES daughters in every group of 1,000 DES women might get vaginal cancer, an estimate that is considerably higher than the current widely accepted statistic of no more than 1.4 DES daughters in every 1,000. There were widespread fears that a cancer epidemic was on the way. "We had to calm things down," one government task force member told me.

Although initial findings soon indicated that the cancer risk for those exposed *in utero* was substantially lower than feared, it was difficult to counteract the panic that mushroomed everywhere. No single word in the American medical vocabulary is more frightening than "cancer," and DES had been firmly associated with a type of cancer that struck young girls just as they were starting their lives.

But there was also reluctance on the part of the government to acknowledge fully the extent of the DES phenomenon—possibly because some people inside federal offices were concerned about a cancer epidemic, possibly because the government itself had for years approved DES for a wide number of uses, possibly because private companies may have been pressuring officials to downplay the whole thing, fearing legal repercussions.

One example of the government's calming effort was a 1976 statement from the National Cancer Institute. After stating that DES had been widely used in pregnancy, it added: "Later studies disclosed that the administration of DES during pregnancy was less effective than initially thought." But since there never were any controlled studies after 1953 showing that it *was* effective—and all the pro-DES studies before 1953 could be faulted on procedural or other grounds—there was no basis for making that statement. Besides, effectiveness wasn't the issue. Side effects were the issue.

The DES task force report, which received widespread publicity, stated that the cancer incidence was quite low, and it correctly articulated many of the concerns that more recent research has borne out— among them, for example, concerns about reproductive problems in men and women and the need for constant monitoring. It stated that physicians and clinics have a professional and ethical responsibility to notify patients of their DES exposure, of the task force's conclusions, and of the need for follow-up care. It said that the use of oral contraceptives and postmenopausal replacement estrogens by DES-exposed women, "though not contraindicated, must be viewed in a prudent fashion, and the decision to use them made only after careful consideration of alternative methods, patient preference, and medical judgment."

The report did have a calming effect on the general public and on the DES-exposed individuals most or exclusively concerned about cancer. But it did little to assuage the anger people felt as day by day, month by month, year by year, they began to discover other problems within their own bodies associated with DES use.

Unfortunately, recent requests from participating centers in the DESAD project for more money to continue research have been denied or cut back altogether, which means that getting the whole DES story out will be more difficult than ever.

One of the most frustrating problems DES-exposed people have is finding out definitely whether they are exposed or not. Some can't get medical recordds at all, at other times medical people lie or evade the issue, while still other patients get their medical records and there is no record of their having taken anything during pregnancy, although they have specific recollections of taking *some* pills on a regular basis.

The task force report recommended that physicians notify all patients of their exposure and recommended also that the federal government begin a public information campaign—a campaign that was later hampered by a lack of money so severe that printed publications on DES sat stacked in warehouses for lack of postage.

There is probably nothing that would catch a patient's eye more than a notice or a phone call from her physician, not to mention hearing that the contact was being made at federal suggestion. But this was virtually never done. One doctor put it this way: "At the time of the task force, local doctors cooperating with them were having no trouble in finding a thousand DES-exposed mothers. Think of what they might have found if they worked at it full time! Our medical malpractice insurance costs were going up then—sometimes they doubled or tripled overnight. We were all terrified of lawsuits. It would be impossible to show that we hadn't been acting in accordance with the best medical care at the time, but even going through a lawsuit is bad for your reputation and your own standing with your peers. A lawsuit takes you away from the office, so you can't treat patients, but you've still got your own overhead and nurses' salaries to pay. That's why there was such reluctance."

According to a still-unreleased federal government report, prepared as a part of the DESAD project, private physicians in some parts of the country were flatly refusing to cooperate with the federal investigators.

The critical report read: ". . . some physicians in Houston are no longer willing to cooperate with Baylor [one of the DESAD centers]. . . . Initially these physicians assured our center that we could examine all the DES-exposed who were located . . . [then] they decided for reasons of their own that they did not want their patients examined at the DES clinic . . . Some of the private physicians have discouraged their private patients from returning to our clinic, feeling they can provide as adequate a follow-up exam." This reluctance within parts of the medical community itself to cooperate with federal health officials—who promised anonymity and protection of specific data—was omitted from the final DES task force report.

Shortly after the 1971 Herbst, Ulfelder, Poskanzer report, seven medical and health-care professionals at the University of Pennsylvania School of Medicine began to locate doctors in the Philadelphia area who might have used DES in their medical practices. According to a report on the project published in the *American Journal of Obstetrics and Gynecology,* 678 physicians were sent letters offering free expert assistance in reviewing their records in an attempt to find DES-exposed people. Only one-third of the total, 216 doctors, even bothered to respond to the letter, and 155 of these said they had used DES. Of this number only 6 desired assistance, while half indicated they wanted no help at all. One-third claimed they had reviewed or would review their own records. The authors of the paper called the 30 percent response rate "disappointing."

There are other expressions of an attitude some physicians have toward patients, which surfaced in the DES controversy. In the June 23, 1980, issue of *Medical World News,* a *Newsweek* type of magazine for physicians, columnist Hans Neumann, M.D., wrote a column entitled, "Patients Have the Right Not to Know." In the article, which dealt in part with the DES-exposed population, he wrote:

I question the intensive search for all DES-exposed persons. An HEW task force demanded that all five to six million such women plus their offspring be traced and notified that they had been exposed to DES. A campaign through the media did an admirable job of alerting the public. But to call it imperative for all involved persons to be sought out and informed of their risk exceeds the bounds of freedom of choice.

Surely those who wish to know about their DES exposure should be given all the data if records still exist. But if others prefer *not* to know, they should have that option. Our current preoccupation with patients' rights should also include the right not to know.

In a 10-year period, perhaps one or two in 10,000 DES daughters develop cancer, while 60 of them are killed in car crashes and many more are maimed, without anticipatory anxiety. Not even a tenth of those who took DES can be located and notified. Thus nine-tenths remain unaware, enjoying themselves to the limit of their capacity for a good life. Most of them will never develop disorders. If problems develop, they usually come to attention in routine examinations or because of symptoms . . . The DES crusade is paralleled by a search for all those who years ago had superficial irradiation for acne . . . Needlessly destroying a patient's emotional balance, his optimism, and his defense mechaniam of denial—unless there are sound reasons to do so—can be more damaging than the disease itself. We can't continue to press the alarm button without knowing that benefits will result.

I asked Neumann, who is director of preventive medicine for the New Haven, Connecticut, department of health, if he still maintained these views. He said he did. "They're much better off not knowing. Of course they should be told if they ask, but if they don't request it, why tell them? Many mothers say to me they don't want to upset their children. If they have regular check-ups they can find out if there are problems. If they have reproductive problems, there's not much that can be done anyway. I don't think my views are popular among doctors. The great vogue now is for truth, regardless of harm."

DES is still approved by the FDA as an estrogen replacement for a number of conditions in postmenopausal women. It is not approved for use as a morning-after pill, although it is still reportedly used that way. It is not approved for the suppression of breast milk after delivery, although thousands of prescriptions are written for its use that way. And it is not approved for use as a drug to stop young men from masturbating, although it has been used that way for more than twenty years in the state of Maryland.

Reporter Margaret Engel of the Washington *Post* reported in November of 1981 that Ruth Baldwin, M.D., director of the University of Maryland's Clinic for Exceptional Children, had been giving DES to more than fifty mentally retarded young men for at least twenty years in an effort to keep them from masturbating in public. The theory apparently was that DES would "feminize" the young men, stop their desire to masturbate, and in controlling that behavior make it possible for them to attend public school classes without incident. Some of the young men developed large breasts. According to a second article Engel published, Baldwin said she would continue giving DES to the young men even if her state bosses refused to peremit her to do so. Mentally handicapped people who have such so-called antisocial conduct can usually be patiently taught not to conduct themselves that way, according to authorities in the field. Baldwin did not return a call to her office.

Since they are doubtful of getting straight answers from the medical profession and anticipate only sluggish responses from health bureaucracies, people wanting information about DES turn to other consumers, people they meet, people they read about, people who answer the phones at consumer groups and health clinics. Phyllis Wetherill receives dozens of letters every month from people seeking information from her DES Registry. When she sends out her newsletters or other documents, she does so in envelopes labeled "Registry," because, she said, some people still feel there is a stigma attached to being DES-exposed, and often they don't want others in their family to know about the information they are seeking.

I asked Dolores Wallgren, vice-president of DES Action, National and head of the group's Washington, D.C., area office, about her experiences as a DES consumer advocate. We talked in the one room of a Montgomery County, Maryland, school they used as their headquarters. "A man rushed in here once wanting information on sons, and then ran out again without giving his name as soon as he got it. DES daughters tell me they hide information we give them so their in-laws and grandparents won't see it. I know a daughter whose father is a pharmacist who filled her mother's presecription for DES. She's afraid to tell him she knows he filled it, and she fears he knows and is hiding it from her. I go into supermarkets wearing our button, which says *Ask Your Mother*. People I don't know are constantly coming up to me, saying 'I'm a DES mother' or 'I'm a DES daughter.'

"People call up, they won't give their names, they demand to know everything we know, but they won't send us any donations to help with our work. Like most consumer groups, we're always hurting for money. We'll ask for support of legislation we want passed, and sometimes they're not interested. They want to find out about the risks, about cancer, and that's it."

Sometimes she takes a stack of telephone messages home with her and calls from there. "The phone bill can be enormous, but it's sort of my contribution. Sometimes I'm on the phone, it seems like twenty-four hours a day. They tell us stories, stories you can't prove but you know are true—the doctor who said his records had been destroyed by a flood, but his office is on the seventh floor of an office building. The fires that only touched some records and not others. Every time there is some public announcement, or a TV show, we're inundated with requests for information. After the *Lou Grant* show had a DES segment, we were swamped. I was in a seminar in Baltimore, and later the phone never stopped ringing. We mailed out two hundred pamphlets in a day. So many daughters say, 'My mother just took vitamins,' but they have adenosis or structural problems. Women don't trust their doctors on this, they call us for a second opinion. 'Is a Pap smear adequate?' 'Will my daughter ever have babies?' We try to help, we have a referral list of doctors in the area who are interested in DES, both for daughters and sons."

Like others in the field, the catchers in the rye for people falling through the system, the burden is sometimes overwhelming. "I'm able to have a good cry now and then—that's the only way to keep going. At a meeting recently two young girls came in. One of them stood up to speak. She said her mother had had two big problems with her. One was that she had been born with mental retardation and the other was that she had been exposed to DES. She spoke eloquently and clearly—and frankly, that just about did it for me."

17
DES AND THE LAW

One day in 1976 Judith Sindell went in to see her boss, a Los Angeles attorney, and in so doing opened up an entirely new era in American product-liability law.

"Before she came in here I had never even heard of DES," her boss, Jason Brent, said in an interview. "I didn't know what it was."

Sindell told Brent that she had been exposed to DES *in utero* and that now, as a young woman of childbearing years, she suffered from vaginal and cervical lesions, adenosis, and a cancerous bladder tumor, which had been removed.

"She said she wanted to sue," he recalled. He agreed to look into it.

There are no courts of morality or ethics in this country, no tribunal of wise elders who pronounce judgments on the daily conduct of others. There are only courts of law, where judges strictly measure certain activities against existing laws and decide whether actions are legal or not, whether one person is harmed by another's actions.

Because there is almost no other way to get "justice"—the concept that embodies a sense of what is absolutely right—people who feel they have been harmed go to court. They sue. They ask the legal system—represented by a judge or a jury—to make the finding that they were harmed and then to undo the harm by making them whole again.

In criminal cases, when a person is robbed or physically injured, society as a whole is hurt and public prosecutors representing "the people" go into court and charge the accused with a crime. The penalty upon conviction can be jail.

In civil cases, an individual or organization sues, claiming that it alone was hurt by another individual or group. In some cases an individual might claim that others in his situation were also hurt. A judge or jury is asked to decide. The punishment is often financial.

One branch of civil law is the product-liability field. When a person claims to be injured by a product, either a lawnmower or an airplane, he sues the manufacturer for damages. In the arcane language of the court, he "prays" for damages to compensate him for his suffering.

What has happened in the DES phenomenon is that people who feel they have been hurt by the drug filed billions of dollars worth of lawsuits in the 1970s, lawsuits that will not be resolved until well into the 1980s or 1990s. By virtue of the concepts involved and the widespread nature of society's exposure to DES, new legal doctrines have been developed that will shape the way courts—and society—view similar cases for decades to come. Arguing those cases for the next decade will be a floating cadre of lawyers on both sides of the issue, some of whom take nothing else but DES cases, some of whom see the issue as an extension of consumer rights, women's rights, or as yet another case of corporate manipulation of consumer needs. The DES bar has become a mini-industry, complete with its own magazine, annual meetings, and everything except uniforms.

Often (surprisingly so for a profession in which "courtroom gray" can refer both to the color of clothing and an emotional attitude) passions run very hot indeed. San Francisco attorney Nancy Hersh, who has filed dozens of cases on behalf of people exposed to DES, once cornered a drug company attorney in a hallway and accused him of representing "murderers." The attorney replied that he was representing a client who had made a legal drug. Russel H. Beatie, Jr., an outside lawyer for Eli Lilly & Company, from the Wall Street law firm of Dewey, Ballantine, Bushby, Palmer & Wood, said he hoped a proposed interview with me would go well so that "after the fact I won't be pissed off at you and want to drop a grenade in your shorts." I was willing to take the chance, but we never had the interview.

Judith Sindell's case has not even come to trial, and yet her name has been inscribed in the legal history books. After she typed her own lawsuit, Jason Brent filed it, on August 2, 1976, on her behalf as well as on behalf of other unnamed DES daughters, in the Superior Court of Los Angeles, the trial court level for the state. The defendants were Abbott Laboratories, E. R. Squibb, Eli Lilly, and other named and unnamed drug manufacturers.

Like other DES-exposed people, she could prove her mother had taken the drug but not who had made the specific product her mother took. In many cases that would have been enough to get the case thrown out of court: if you can't say who harmed you, you can't sue. But DES was different; it was made with the same unpatented formula by a wide variety of companies that had pooled their resources at government request and used the same studies and research in getting FDA approval back in the 1940s.

Attorney Brent alleged, among other things, negligence, breach of warranty, and fraud. The drug companies objected on standard grounds—no specific maker, no lawsuit—but after the California Supreme Court heard the arguments, it agreed, in March of 1980, that Sindell should get her day in court. The drug companies appealed, but seven months later the U.S. Supreme Court declined to look at the issue. History had been made, and a new era in product-liability law had come into being.

The California Supreme Court stated in an opinion written by Justice Stanley Mosk:

> In our contemporary complex industrialized society, advances in science and technology create fungible [identically produced] goods which may harm consumers and which cannot be traced to any specific producer. The response of the courts can be either to adhere rigidly to prior doctrines . . . or to fashion remedies to meet these changing needs.
>
> [The] plaintiff is not at fault in failing to provide evidence of causation, and although the absence of such evidence is not attributable to the defendants either, their conduct in marketing a drug the effects of which are delayed for many years played a significant role in creating the unavailability of proof. . . .
>
> The manufacturer is in the best position to discover and guard against defects in its products and to warn of harmful effects; thus, holding it liable for defects and failure to warn of harmful effects will provide an incentive to product safety.

Since it was not known which company had made the DES Sindell's mother had taken, the court ruled that each defendant could be held responsible according to his share of the total DES market. Thus if a company made 50 percent of all DES, it would be liable for 50 percent of the damages. However, the court did not provide a guide for determining their respective shares of the market.

DES, which had seemingly changed the course of medical history by offering a cure for miscarriages, had thus changed the course of legal history by figuring in a decision allowing people to sue even if they didn't know the maker of a commonly marketed product that hurt them.

The Sindell theory may have an application in a wide variety of other fields—chemical waste cases, asbestos cases—in which the product is made by various manufacturers from a common formula. Other state courts, including Michigan, have already handed down similar rulings. State court rulings can be appealed to higher courts within the state or to the U.S. Supreme Court. So far, only the Sindell case has made it all the way to the top.

Judith Sindell's case isn't expected to come to trial for another few years, but the damages involved if she wins could be enormous. Attorney Brent asked for actual damages of one million dollars for her and ten million dollars against each of the defendants.

But Brent also filed the case as a class action, claiming that what had happened to her had happened to a great many other women, that Sindell is just one of the class of women affected by DES. A judge must decide if indeed there are other people whose interests should be represented in the case. If the matter is certified as a class-action case, with an estimated three hundred thousand DES women in California, the money damages could be astronomical. "It could be the most important class-action case in the last fifty years," Brent said. "There could be damages of more than one billion dollars in California alone. These women have been harmed, and I've got a tiger by the tail. The attitude of the drug company lawyers is just 'Grind the bastard down'—and I'm the bastard."

Robert Dickson (a partner in the Los Angeles firm of Haight, Dickson, Brown & Bonesteel and head of national litigation for E. R. Squibb & Sons) is Brent's opposite number in the Sindell case. He doesn't quite see it that way. "The ruling was about the best we could hope for at this stage," he said. "I talked to the law clerks at the U.S. Supreme Court after the justices declined to review the California decision, and they indicated the Supreme Court would review the whole case after the issues have been tried." (Craig Diamond, the DES son with testicular cancer, once worked in Dickson's firm.)

The issues of negligence, breach of warranty, and fraud in the Sindell case will be even more complex than they are in other DES cases. Although she had a cancerous bladder tumor, which was removed, her fertility has not been impaired: several years ago Judith Sindell had a baby. But in view of all that has been learned about DES exposure, especially the potential long-range effects, the court will have to decide whether she was hurt from her DES exposure or whether she has been hurt by the fear that something may happen to her later in life.

In Massachusetts the nation's first court-certified product-liability class action case—a DES case—seeks multimillion-dollar damages on similar grounds. The suit (known as *Payton* v. *Abbott Laboratories* et. al.) represents nearly four thousand women in Massachusetts who claim to have suffered noncancerous physical and emotional injuries because of their DES exposure. The suit also seeks the establishment of free screening clinics for DES-exposed people in Massachusetts, as well as an insurance fund in case cancer later develops.

In a third-floor walk-up office off Harvard Square, where plants hang in mullioned windows, attorneys Jeanne Baker and David Fine are continuing a conceptual case developed by Harvard law professor David Rosenberg: Do people have a right to sue for emotional stress and anxiety caused by the statistical probability that they will suffer harm in the future? In effect, Baker and Fine are asking for damages for women who at the moment have no demonstrable physical harm but have reason to fear that they may have in the future.

In response, attorneys from the Boston firm of Goodwin, Procter & Hoar, led by Marshall Simons, have argued that the plaintiffs have no right to sue, because without DES they would never have been born. Papers filed in the case state that the defendants will show at the trial that the "same DES which plaintiffs allege has harmed them, or may harm them, enabled [them] to be born in the first place." If that happens, it would mark the first time since the 1950s that anyone had tried to show that DES actually worked.

In Chicago a DES case raised ethical questions about the ways certain medical studies were conducted, and by virtue of the case's outcome, the way they will probably never be conducted again in the future. Three women who were part of the famous Dieckmann study in the 1950s—the double-blind study that showed DES was ineffective in preventing miscarriages—sued the University of Chicago for battery (the unauthorized touching of another person) and related charges, claiming they were given DES without their knowledge or consent. The three women were Phyllis Wetherill, former congresswoman Patsy Mink; and Gladys Engel Lang, a professor of sociology in New York. They claimed that the university essentially lied to them by saying they were taking "vitamin pills" and by delaying five years before telling them of their DES exposure, even after the 1971 cancer report had been issued.

Phyllis Wetherill's pretrial testimony was compelling enough. After her daughter, Rachel, heard a news report about the DES-cancer link, Phyllis contacted the University of Chicago and asked a representative if she'd been part of that study or had been given DES. She said she was told no. "We were living in Los Angeles at the time and there was a DES clinic at UCLA. Rachel could have gone there for a checkup."

The court records state that the University of Chicago's Lying-In Hospital (where Rachel had been born) later confirmed her mother's DES exposure, but only after it had received a government grant to do so. "Once again it all comes down to money," Phyllis Wetherill said. In defending itself in court papers, the University of Chicago denied it had acted improperly and said that women coming into the Chicago Lying-In clinic were told verbally what they would be taking. Dieckmann's original 1953 paper states that each woman was told the pills "would cause no harm to her or the fetus."

Although the legal issue was battery, the case was redolent of the issue of "informed consent," a legal and social concept that requires medical professionals to tell a patient explicitly everything that is about to happen (including all potential aftereffects) and then make sure that person fully understands what has been said. In today's medical world informed consent is documented by a signed consent form, although that was not the custom back in the 1950s when the Dieckmann study was conducted.

So the Chicago case asked: Did the women know exactly what they were taking? Had they been informed of all the medical ramifications? Had they signed a consent form? Had they been fully advised of all the risks? Had they been unlawfully touched, or battered, by the university? The suit was tried in Chicago's Federal Court in February of 1981. William B. Schultz and John Cary Sims, the attorneys from the Ralph Nader-founded Public Citizen's Litigation Group, which was representing the three women, called more than a dozen witnesses. The university then began its own defense, but midway through the trial it agreed to an out-of-court settlement.

The school agreed to pay $225,000 to the three women, and it also agreed to provide medical examinations to the women and men exposed to DES during their mothers' participation in the Dieckmann study and to notify the nearly 1,000 people born to women in the study about the availability of treatment. This last point is significant. Although the suit as it was tried was not a class-action suit, the university was to act as if it were, and would provide treatment for everyone involved in the Dieckmann study, not just for these women and their children. The university did not admit any wrongdoing in its actions, and it still faces numerous legal actions brought by daughters of women in the suit, who have sued both the school and the Eli Lilly company.

The University of Chicago was not the only school to give women DES in a controlled study during the 1950s. Among others, Tulane University's Charity Hospital also studied DES, and the principal author of a paper produced there, John Henry Ferguson, also concluded that DES was ineffective in preventing miscarriages. I inquired at the hospital information office whether they had ever notified members of the study group of their DES exposure, but the hospital never responded to my inquiry. Ironically, the woman who took my call, and to whom I wrote a letter, said she was a DES daughter.

Although the Dieckmann study had settled for much of the medical community the question of DES effectiveness, because its conclusions were based on strict objective principles, the controversy that has swirled about its method for choosing people for the study and its informal way of giving them some of the information available have contributed to the widespread practice of seeking informed consent from people participating in medical and clinical studies. The alternative, the medical profession now knows, is to end up in court.

Besides the complex legal and social issues that have not yet come to trial, there have been a number of courtroom confrontations over DES exposure. The drug companies have been found innocent in some of those cases, while other cases have been settled out of court for undisclosed sums. There have also been a number of important verdicts involving young women with clear-cell adenocarcinoma.

On February 11, 1983, Eli Lilly & Company agreed to pay 21-year-old Barbara Watson $250,000 in cash and $30,000 a year for life to settle the suit she had brought against the company. Ms. Watson developed vaginal cancer; her mother had taken DES during pregnancy. The company denied all liability. Her attorney, Washington, D.C. lawyer Aaron M. Levine, said that if Ms. Watson lives another 50 years, the payments will reach an estimated $1.7 million.

One landmark decision was made on March 24, 1982, when a jury in Philadelphia ordered E. R. Squibb & Sons to pay nearly $2.2 million to Judith Axler, whose mother had taken DES made by Squibb during her pregnancy with Judith in 1960. The young woman developed clear-cell cancer, and now, after surgery, is unable to have children. That award is larger than all the other awards in DES cases put together. Judith Axler's lawyer, Herbert F. Kolsby, said that because the product identification was so strong, the jury focused on whether or not the company was negligent in marketing the drug for pregnancy, whether or not it failed to warn of potential dangers, whether or not it was effective, and whether or not it caused cancer, both generally and in Miss Axler's case. The jury decided completely in her favor. They found that the company had been negligent, had failed to warn of dangers, that DES had not been effective as a deterrent to miscarriage, and had caused her cancer. The verdict is expected to be appealed.

The first case won (1979) by a DES-exposed person was brought by Joyce Bichler, whose mother had taken DES during pregnancy. Born in 1954, Bichler subsequently developed vaginal cancer. Although she could not identify the manufacturer, her attorneys (former New York State Supreme Court Justice Leonard Finz and Sybil Schainwald) sued Eli Lilly & Company on the grounds that it had been an early and major manufacturer of the drug and that its representatives had been involved at all stages of getting government approval for the drug for a wide variety of uses. That concept was unique. It worked.

The 1979 trial made reference to a 1978 *Fordham Law Review* article that advanced the new concept of industry-wide, or enterprise, liability, in situations in which an entire industry had produced and marketed an identical product. The jury in the Bichler case was asked seven questions which by their very nature are historic in determining within a legal framework what is proper conduct for a drug company:

"Was DES reasonably safe in the treatment of accidents of pregnancy when it was ingested by [Bichler's] mother in 1953?" The answer was No.

"Was DES a proximate cause of [Bichler's] cancer?" Yes.

"In 1953 when [Bichler's] mother ingested DES, should [Eli Lilly], as a reasonable prudent drug manufacturer, have foreseen that DES might cause cancer in the offspring of pregnant women who took it?" Yes.

"Foreseeing that DES might cause cancer in the offspring of pregnant women who took it, would a reasonably prudent drug manufacturer test it on pregnant mice before marketing it?" Yes.

"If DES had been tested on pregnant mice, would the tests have shown tht DES causes cancer in their offspring?" Yes.

"Would a reasonably prudent drug manufacturer have marketed DES for use in treating accidents of pregnancy at the time it was ingested by [Bichler's] mother if it had known that DES causes cancer in the offspring of pregnant mice?" No.

"Did [Eli Lilly] and other drug manufacturers act in concert with each other in the testing and marketing of DES for use in treating accidents of pregnancy?" Yes.

The six-member jury then awarded Bichler $500,000. The award has been upheld.

Drug company lawyers, led by Lilly, have fought that verdict on a number of grounds: that Lilly had never been identified as the actual maker of the drug Bichler's mother took, that the answers to the questions were not all unanimous (some of them were five-to-one splits in Bichler's favor), and so on. And because of the precedent-setting nature of the case—that one drug company has been held responsible despite a lack of specific proof connecting it to the injury—the case has been on appeal for years, and is expected to be appealed all the way to the U.S. Supreme Court.

Another DES case, this one based on more traditional grounds, was won by a woman with cancer. In 1979 Michigan resident Anne Needham was awarded $800,000 from White Laboratories. The jury ruled that the company had made the DES her mother took, causing Anne Needham's clear-cell vaginal cancer. An appeals court overturned the verdict on technical grounds, and a new trial was scheduled.

Although new medical knowledge has been woven through the lawsuits, it is important to note the differences in approach of the two disciplines. The Herbst paper and others like it have always claimed that DES use by pregnant mothers was "associated" with clear-cell adenocarcinoma in their daughters. The legal forums work on a tighter standard than that: the Bichler jury was asked if DES had been a "proximate [or very near] cause" of Joyce Bichler's cancer, and the verdict, by a five-to-one vote, was that it had been.

Science, then, holds out the possibility that other chemical actions may have caused the cancer, though DES may have initiated the process; the law eliminates most of the middle steps and looks at the cause-and-effect relationship.

DES litigation has almost become an industry in itself. In fighting more than 600 lawsuits brought by more than 6,000 named plaintiffs in more than 40 states, two distinct cadres of lawyers have developed their expertise in the field and have become nationally known as DES plaintiff attorneys or DES defense attorneys. On the plaintiffs' side, the first major DES lawyer was Lawrence S. Charfoos of Detroit, a product-liability attorney who got involved with DES cases in part because so many DES daughters in that area had had partial vaginectomies to eliminate adenosis. The controversial medical procedure was most popular in Detroit, although almost nowhere else.

Charfoos estimates he has invested more than one million dollars in time and money to research the issue. He was the original attorney for Anne Needham, and when attorney Jason Brent needed information for his suit on behalf of Judith Sindell, he used Charfoos' research. (Brent also used the theoretical concepts developed by the Baker and Fine firm in Boston.) Like other lawyers who have developed a specialty in a particular field, Charfoos charges for his expertise: if he simply makes material available to another lawyer, he charges 10 percent of the eventual award, if any. If he directly participates in a case, the fee increases. He also sells copies of his appeals-court brief in his Michigan case on behalf of a woman named Gail Abel, who could not identify the company that made the DES her mother took. The cost for the brief is $100, in order to defray some of his prior costs incurred in having his brief copied. The Charfoos firm is involved in more than 300 cases.

San Francisco attorney Nancy Hersh has used the Charfoos material for her cases, as has Washington trial attorney Aaron M. Levine. In Los Angeles, Roman Silberfeld has handled a number of DES cases, as has Herbert Kolsby in Philadelphia. In Connecticut attorney Michael Koskoff has filed a class action suit on behalf of an estimated 12,000 to 20,-000 Connecticut women exposed to DES whose injuries ranged anywhere from death to fear of the future.

Defending the drug companies are attorneys representing, first, Lilly and Squibb, and through other arrangements, the smaller firms as well. Russel H. Beattie, Jr., in New York, Lane Bauer in Kansas City, and Richard Heafy in Oakland, California, fly incessantly around the country on behalf of Eli Lilly. When the case of Judith Axler was heard in Philadelphia (in March 1982) Robert L. Dickson of Los Angeles handled the Squibb defense. Opposing him was Kolsby. They had previously opposed each other in another case against Squibb. Dickson won that one, and the charges were dismissed against Squibb; he lost in the Axler case, when the jury returned what is in effect a $2.2 million verdict.

The defense attorneys are from the absolute top of the market:

Dewey Ballantine in New York; Hogan and Hartson in Washington; Murphy and Mitchell in Boston; Adams, Duque, Hazeltine in Los Angeles; Lord, Bissell, Brook in Chicago; and so on.

The DES lawyers on both sides of the fence can read about themselves and their cases in the *DES Litigation Reporter*, a $600-a-year summary of DES cases published twice monthly by Andrews Publications, Inc., in suburban Philadelphia. The publication averages 66 pages per issue, and it took three complete issues to publish the list of all 400 lawsuits against Eli Lilly & Company.

The volume of cases has gotten so great that when retired University of Chicago pathologist Edith L. Potter, now eighty-one years old, was deposed recently, more than 100 attorneys in 290 separate cases rented a television studio in Kansas City to watch her tape her answers. The fact that she was permitted to tape her deposition at all, much less have the same videotape recording use in hundreds of different cases, is another sign of how the sheer volume of DES suits is changing the way the law is practiced.

The use of television and electronic technology was virtually pioneered in the DES cases. In Boston, Baker and Fine coordinated the plaintiffs' side in a national mass videotape deposition program so that each of the historic figures in the DES matter could testify once and provide material for use in dozens—or hundreds—of cases. Attorney John F. Triggs (of Slade Pellman & Biehl, in Manhattan, which represents Emons Industries, Inc., now a parent company to a former DES manufacturer) was one of the lawyers at the Kansas City deposition. However, instead of getting as close to the witness as possible, Triggs went to the back of the studio to watch the testimony on the TV monitor. "That's what the jury is going to see," he said. Triggs also thinks the increasing use of television production techniques in trials may lead some lawyers to take acting lessons, or, at the very least, figure out how to look good on camera. "If you don't know what to do with your hands in front of a camera, you better learn," he said.

How much do lawyers—on both sides—get? Attorneys for plaintiffs—the people bringing the suits—will receive as much as one-third or more of any award, when it is finally issued after all appeals. Attorneys for drug companies can bill at two hundred dollars or more per hour, and the clock starts running with every phone call. One inside attorney says that in one three-month period Eli Lilly paid one million dollars to just one of the law firms representing it. He says he saw the bill. Lilly declines to discuss specifics.

In our system of law, any individual or company accused of wrong-doing has the absolute right to fight that accusation, or conviction, as far and as long and as hard as possible. Drug companies argue that the concepts of the 1950s shouldn't be applied to the 1980s; that there was no way for them to have known about the hazards of DES; that it was tested by the best scientists; that the statute of limitations protects them. (Statute of limitations means that lawsuits can be brought only a few years after a pereson is harmed by a product—for example, a few years after a mother took DES, and not twenty years later when her daughter gets cancer or finds she can't get pregnant.)

But there is also an economic factor that goes beyond DES. DES is a generic drug. Currently there are 1,862 generic drugs made by only one manufacturer, and 4,081 generic drugs made by a variety of manufacturers, according to the Generic Pharmaceutical Manufacturers Association. The *Physicians' Desk Reference,* which contains listings supplied by manufacturers for all drugs sold, has 31 pages of single-spaced lines listing thousands of generic products. Generic drugs are produced by many manufacturers according to one common formula—just as DES was produced. The field of general drugs is also growing rapidly. From 1977 to 1979, when the total pharmaceutical market expanded by 10 percent, generic drugs increased in sales by 12.6 percent. In 1970, 7 percent of all prescriptions were written for generic drugs, but by 1979 that figure had risen to 14 percent. Four out of five generic drugs were made by the same major manufacturer who are involved in the DES litigation.

If the DES cases set a precedent, then any future problems with generic drugs will be seen in the same light, with millions of dollars worth of claims filed against the companies by consumers who now have the legal tools to fight them. Large manufacturers of generic drugs often fear that precedent-setting lawsuits will be lost by small drug companies that made products identical to their own. Sometimes the big legal guns from the major companies take over the court cases of the smaller companies. The tiny Carnrick Laboratories was once sued in a DES case in New Jersey, but its defense was handled by Russel H. Beatie, Jr., one of Eli Lilly's leading outside attorneys. The case was settled before a verdict was reached.

In addition, if drug companies are ordered by juries to pay huge sums of money to people damaged years later by their products, who actually pays? The drug companies' insurance carriers. But do they pay according to the amount of coverage in effect thirty years earlier, when the drug was used, or according to the amount of coverage in effect today? Within the multibillion-dollar insurance industry this is a major question. The insurance companies would like to pay at the low rate of coverage in effect decades ago, amounts so small they look like today's auto-policy coverage. But the drug companies would like them to pay at the rates of today, which are in line with the size of awards juries today are giving. The issue is being hotly debated across the country, and at least one lawsuit has been filed by a drug company against an insurance carrier because of it. If the insurance companies charge the drug companies more for coverage in an era of large settlements in regard to a generic drug such as DES, it is more than possible that the drug companies will pass that increase along to the consumer in the form of higher prices for drugs.

What about the small drug companies that did market a drug like DES but also get caught up in lawsuits involving generic products? In cases in which no specific manufacturer is known, should they pay as much in damages as a giant company, which might be theoretically better able to handle the burden? "No," says drug company attorney John F. Triggs, whose client, he said, made less than one-half of 1 percent of all DES produced in this country. "I think Sindell is right: the plaintiff can recover from a defendant in accordance with the share of the market the defendant had. Otherwise the little defendant is going to have a judgment exceeding his share of the market." That would not be fair, Triggs said. "Five years ago I remember everyone saying [the] Sindell [decision] was crazy. Now it's in place. Everyone copied everyone else's information, back then. [DES] was as common as aspirin." That type of talk pits the little drug companies against the big ones, and in fact Triggs and other lawyers have started to file what are called third-party cases against the larger drug companies, trying to get them named as codefendants in original suits.

To stay out of the courthouse, go to the statehouse. That has been the latest development in the DES phenomenon. In an attempt to circumvent the implications of the Sindell decision, legislators friendly to the drug industry have introduced bills that would require people to identify positively the maker of the product that hurt them—legislation that would overturn Sindell.

In 1980 and 1981 that legislation was introduced in the California legislature. It was defeated only after aggressive lobbying by consumer groups and, not insignificantly, representatives of trial lawyers who handle DES cases. Other state legislators have seen the same thing. In California a political lobbying firm hired by a major DES maker put out the word that there was a minimum of fifty thousand dollars available to make sure the legislation passed. The money was to be funneled through an over-all industry group so it could not be traced to the company. The money was spent, but the legislation failed.

There are also efforts to create the same kind of anti-Sindell legislation on the national level. In Washington a proposed bill supported by industry and being considered in both the House and Senate would set up a federal law standardizing all state product-liability laws, and require that people who sue for damages be able to identify the specific company that allegedly harmed them. The first public hearings on the bill took place on March 9, 1982, before Wisconsin Republican Senator Robert W. Kasten, Jr. The large hearing room in the Russell Office Building had a standing-room-only crowd of lawyers and representatives of such trade groups as the U.S. Chamber of Commerce, the National Association of Manufacturers, the Chemical Manufacturers Associations, and dozens more. There was so much corporate interest in the hearing that well-heeled lawyers and women lobbyists in fur coats had to wait outside in the hallway until there was room for them inside. In the best Washington tradition, more than a hundred and fifty businesses and trade associations have joined together to form their own lobbying group, the Product Liability Alliance. Representatives of many of the groups testified.

Testifying on behalf of consumers were Sidney M. Wolfe, M.D., and Allen Greenberg, from the Public Citizens Health Research Group. In their statements they pointed out that there are three ways of regulating corporate behavior, "all of which are essential in order to minimize the amount of damage done to people by dangerous products." First is public information through package labeling and new reports; second is government regulation itself, through such agencies as the FDA; the third are lawsuits in which, "it is said, if there is an injury, there should be a remedy." With current government cutbacks on public information, as well as a trend toward deregulation of all government processes, the process of legal action for consumers is crucial, they said. "If anything, something should be done to make it easier, not more difficult, for people to get compensated in product-liability cases," Wolfe and Greenberg stated. "At a time when the sentiment in [the Senate] is to leave traditional state functions to the states—the essence of Federalism—it borders on the hypocritical to propose that Congress should dictate to the state courts the rules these courts must apply in product-liability cases."

Sindell-type decisions, which allow injured people to sue all manufacturers of identical products even when they cannot identify the specific manufacturer, frighten industry, insurance and legal representatives. In fact, drug industry attorney Russel H. Beatie, Jr., told a judge in a 1978 DES trial in New Jersey federal court: "This case represents a threat to the continued existence of the pharmaceutical industry as we know it in this country."

The law has not had significant impact on drug companies alone. Some DES-exposed people have seen it as a vehicle not only for righting the wrong they feel was done to them but as a way of getting rid of enormous anger at having had their lives damaged by DES. Boston psychiatrist Roberta Apfel, M.D., said that vastly more women agreed to participate in the Massachusetts class-action suit than came in for examinations at free local clinics. Several women I interviewed were perfectly willing to be identified and quoted at length in this book until they decided to file lawsuits; their attorneys suggested that their published stories might be harmful to the case, so they asked that the information be deleted.

Not to be outdone, an attorney representing DES-exposed people offered to give me copies of publicly available court papers if I would share all my research with his clients. I declined. Two lawyers representing DES women literally "ambulance-chased" as they sought clients for their suits. They went to meetings of DES Action groups and talked about the money that could result from successful suits. One of them later tried to drop a client from a lawsuit when he determined she did not have as strong a case as he had originally thought.

The impact of the unprecedented number of lawsuits in the DES field, and the hostility that many of those suits has engendered, can be seen everywhere. Manufacturers are required to file a statement, called a 10-K statement, with the Securities and Exchange Commission (SEC) listing all outstanding legal actions against them that could affect the value of their publicly traded stock. In the 10-K statement filed by Lilly in 1975 the company stated: "It is believed that during the late 1940s and early 1950s the Company was a major manufacturer of DES." But then the multimillion-dollar suits began being regularly filed against the firm, whose 10-K statement for 1982 reads: "The Company does not know if it was a major manufacturer of DES for use during pregnancy to prevent miscarriage."

Researchers who testify in court are attacked privately by whatever side does not like their testimony. When they refuse to testify at all, they are attacked for that. Several attorneys for DES women have a team of medical specialists to whom they send their clients. They may send them to different doctors until they get the medical opinion that will do them the most good in court.

Going to court can be an ugly, humiliating process for the people who have been grievously hurt by their DES exposure. Cases can take up to a decade to come to trial, with an appeals process lasting years more. Every aspect of the plaintiff's background is scrutinized by drug company lawyers, both in accordance with the standard pretrial practice of finding flaws in the case and (one suspects) to serve as a reminder to others considering suit that a legal proceeding involving potentially millions of dollars is never taken lightly by trial attorneys.

In *Gloria Reid et al.* v. *Eli Lilly et al.*, a case filed by attorney Aaron M. Levine in federal court in the District of Columbia, the drug companies were granted permission to compel all female plaintiffs to reveal the names and addresses of all their sexual partners, "venereal diseases and other diseases," and methods of birth control they had used. The information would be kept sealed—that is, not made a part of the public record. But the women would still have to reveal it.

In another incident in that same case a plaintiff was asked in a deposition about her "vaginal itching," antibiotics taken for strep throat, how many sexual partners she had had, X-rays she may have received, the nature of her dental care, and the name of her dentist. That type of rough questioning is standard in many lawsuits, and is proper under the rules permitting lawyers to obtain all relevant information with which to defend their clients. But it also means the road to judgment will be a rocky one.

Why do they go through it? Some women say they do it to "get even," to assuage the anger and hurt they feel. Some of them say, off the record, that they are interested in the money damages, both as punishment for the drug companies and for the money itself. But most say that they want to use the vehicle of the law and the court system to make sure that what happened to them will never happen to anyone again, ever.

18

THE FUTURE

Could it happen again?

Could there be another wonder drug developed for one purpose, used for another, tested by the best people, marketed by the leading companies, approved by all the government agencies, answering a desperate social need—which later produces nightmares?

Yes.

Standards are what we say they are. Caution is the invisible buffer between advancing technology and common sense. Risk is the chasm we willingly leap, attempting to go from desire to result.

Diethylstilbestrol—DES—was thought to be the perfect answer from those who say the modern world is perfect, with built-in safety factors to eliminate disaster. Use DES only for people with repeated miscarriages? Only in small doses? Why hold back on something like this? Give it to people who *might* have miscarriages; give it in large doses, small doses—everybody knows the placenta will protect the fetus. DES failed because of its own built-in errors—human errors that no system can prevent.

If we put our faith in fail-safe systems, as surely as the DES-exposed people in this book have testified, we will fail too.

The human body has 200 billion cells; a newborn has 350 separate bones and blood cells so small that only now we know they measure .002 millimeters thick. To say the body runs like clockwork is to flatter the clock. To say we know how it works is to admit we are at the base of the mountain, looking up. We know more—much more—than we did, but we don't know everything. Perhaps we never will. Which is not to say that we should shuck off our clothes, run wild in the heather, live off roots and nuts, and insist that everything that passes our lips and enters our bodies be certified pure and natural and untouched by human hands or man-made chemicals.

But one of the many lessons of the DES experience is that the balance was shattered between a new product our technology-proud society developed and the impact of its side effects so many years later. Some people are still stunned by the time gap. For almost the first time we saw a generation grow up between a drug's action and its later impact. Was it a mistake when the best medical minds used the drug for one purpose, putting aside its potential side effects? It happened all the time. No one ever thought X-ray radiation and toxic chemicals were good for people—it was just thought that they couldn't do any harm. The leading drug companies didn't think they were committing crimes when they sold DES; they certainly didn't set out to disrupt the lives of those still unborn. But in acting only within the law, without taking further moral responsibility, in ignoring the conflicting signs and the warning signals, in letting consumers take the risk, they were permitted by society to act legally but irresponsibly. Legal irresponsibility—that is the least of what happened.

A miscarriage in the family? A terrible event, an event of tears and anguish. But a common event—20 out of every 100 pregnancies will end that way—but common enough so that 17 of those 20 women will eventually have babies. A love of children spurred the desire; a desire to heal, to cure the hurt caused by miscarriage spurred the prescription; an interest in helping and in making profits spurred the production; and DES became a widely used drug, a seed planted in society which would bear its bitter fruit a generation later. Perhaps we all share some innocence. Perhaps we all share some blame.

Is today any different?

Look in your medicine cabinet right now, or downstairs beside the kitchen sink. In nearly every American household today one can find a bottle of aspirin. Fine for headaches—although significantly, scientists are still unsure exactly how it works. But for pregnant women? "Premature infants whose mothers ingested aspirin in the week prior to delivery had a significantly increased risk of intracranial hemorrhage. In light of this finding, maternal aspirin use in the last trimester of pregnancy must be considered highly questionable and probably inappropriate," according to a report by Carole M. Rumack, M.D.

A friendly drink during pregnancy? A cup of coffee? "Maternal smoking and caffeine use have various deleterious effects on fetal and neonatal development and outcome. With determination and compassion, physicians should urge women not to smoke during pregnancy," reported Loretta P. Finnegan, M.D.

Indeed, the FDA has now required the manufacturers of nonprescription over-the-counter drugs to print a warning urging pregnant women to consult a physician before using the products.

For years vitamins were routinely prescribed during pregnancy to help the mother stay healthy, which would in turn help the baby. Doctors gave free samples, patients bought their own. But too many vitamins can adversely affect the physical and mental development of the fetus. This was known; this was ignored.

In the area of prescription drugs, Bendectin, the only government-approved drug used to combat "morning sickness" during pregnancy, may be linked to birth defects in some children whose mothers took it; the U.S. distributor says it is safe. A warning was added to the label in 1982 stating that high dosages of the drug may cause birth deformities in test animals. But should a pregnant woman risk the trade-off between relief from morning sickness and possible harm to her unborn child?

Thalidomide is the prescription drug most often mentioned in the same breath with DES. It was prescribed as a tranquilizer, and some babies born to women who took it did not have arms or legs. "In the wake of the thalidomide and diethylstilbestrol (DES) tragedies," reported Hugh R. K. Barber, M.D., "both the medical profession and the public emerged newly knowledgeable and vigilant. But the effects of drug therapy in pregnancy are often unpredictable, and much remains to be learned. It is sobering to realize that the incidence of birth defects has not decreased notably in recent years . . . Obstetricians and pediatricians must redouble their efforts to ensure that disasters will not occur."

Rumack, Finnegan, and Barber spoke at a May 1981 symposium on drug therapy and pregnancy held in New York.

How to be sure?

Thalidomide was given to laboratory test rats. They were fine; their offspring were fine. The drug was widely used in Europe, hardly at all in the U.S., because an American FDA official wanted more information. That was in the 1950s. But not for another thirty years would the *mechanism* of thalidomide's horrible impact be known: "The human liver converts it into a derivative called arene oxide, which is toxic to fetal cells. In contrast, the rat's liver when processing the drug, does not produce this dangerous metabolite," a research team headed by Gary B. Gordon told the National Academy of Sciences in 1981.

The thalidomide disaster showed that even animal testing could be inadequate for determining the possible impact of a drug given to people. But recently, because of the DES experience, a number of researchers asked themselves if it would be possible to grow human tissue in animal hosts, subject that human tissue to a drug, and then see what happened to the human tissue. In that way the impact of a drug on people could be determined without subjecting people to the drug itself, and the problem that arose in the thalidomide tests—experiments using animals which metabolized thalidomide differently from people—could be avoided.

Stanley J. Robboy, M.D. (a Harvard pathologist who is also a coprincipal investigator of the DESAD team), and Gerald R. Cunha, Ph.D., thought that athymic "nude" mice—a new strain of test mice that do not have a thymus gland and so do not have an immune system—might provide a good host for human fetal tissue. The normal strains of experimental mice would naturally reject the human tissue implants and thus make testing impossible.

A colony of such "nude" mice was maintained in a germ-free incubator environment for two years and then implanted with human tissue. One group of mice was treated with DES, the other was not. The resuslts (published by Robboy, Cunham, and Osamu Taguchi, Ph.D., in the March 1982 issue of *Human Pathology*) show that the DES-exposed human tissue developed anatomical and structural abnormalities similar to those that studies have shown develop in humans subjected during pregnancy to DES. Such tests would not have been possible in the 1930s and 1940s, Robboy said, because the athymic mouse strain was developed only in the 1970s. "We want to sit back and consider where we go from here," Robboy said. Whether such newly available tests will be used by drug companies or required by the federal government as it cuts back on federal safety standards under the Reagan Administration is uncertain.

Pregnancy is not the only time when we take more risks than we have to. For example, Flagyl is a prescription drug made by Searle Pharmaceuticals. It is commonly prescribed for both women and men for *Trichomonas vaginalis* vaginitis infections, which occur in the vagina in women and urinary tract in men. The principal ingredient of Flagyl is metronidazole, a chemical that has been shown to be carcinogenic in mice and rats. The "Warning" section of the package insert for Flagyl correctly states: "Its use, therefore, should be reserved for serious anaerobic infections where, in the judgment of the physician, the benefit outweighs the possible risk."

But women have an alternative to the use of this expensive prescription drug whose main ingredient is carcinogenic in animals: soap and water. In the October 15, 1965, issue of the *American Journal of Obstetrics and Gynecology,* Larry McGowan, M.D., described 94 women who had been relieved of the symptoms within seven days after daily self-cleansing with plain, nonmedicated Ivory or Dial soap. The recurrence rate of the irritation was more than 35 percent for women who did not follow the daily self-cleansing technique, and only 5 percent in the women who did. The 5 percent figure could be due to many factors, including improper bathing techniques, or other types of medical problems, according to one medical figure.

If soap-and-water works for most women, why should all take a risk?

In the March 15–31, 1982, issue of *Ob.Gyn News* there is an article suggesting confusion in the medical community as to whether or not nonmedicated IUDs should be periodically removed for health reasons. More than 2.3 million American women currently wear nonmedicated IUDs, which have been associated with some cases of pelvic inflammatory disease in a number of long-term users. The point is, if there is dispute in the medical community over whether or not an IUD should be periodically removed and replaced, why should women bear the brunt of the confusion?

Oral contraceptives are a constant source of controversy in the medical profession. Their use has been associated with increased risk of heart attacks, strokes, and other problems, especially in older women who smoke, according to an article by Bruce Stadel, M.D., a medical officer with the National Institute of Child Health and Human Development's Contraceptive Development Branch. The precise mechanism for the development of the problems is not known. But why take the risk?

The mother of a friend of mine died from ovarian cancer. My friend's aunt, on her father's side, is currently dying of breast cancer. The estrogen in oral contraceptives has been associated in laboratory animals with breast cancer. In spite of knowing this and my friend's family history, her gynecologist suggested she use oral contraceptives, saying the risk was minimal. She refused. Why take the risk at all?

All of this indicates the interlocking relationships between physicians and their patients. Patients must be responsible for themselves, because history has clearly shown that they cannot necessarily depend on others to do it for them. The legal labyrinth in which drug companies now find themselves because of DES may serve to ensure that they will test their products more carefully. But maybe not: legal costs are tax-deductible, the cost of doing business.

In truth, doctors and consumers have a lot to do with what drug companies make and market. In 1974 Thomas C. Chalmers, M.D., dean of the Mount Sinai School of Medicine in New York, looked at three traditional therapies that were used despite the fact that other, controlled studies had found each of them to be useless, or harmful. One of them was DES. His commonsense conclusion: "Physicians who wish to continue to employ therapies that have been found by peer review to be ineffective, or more toxic than efficacious, should be expected, as in the case of investigative procedures and drugs, to submit their plans to peer review and to obtain truly informed consent from their patients."

DES is not the only drug that didn't work. In 1980 Sidney M. Wolfe, M.D. and members of Public Citizen's Health Research Group published a book called *Pills That Don't Work*, a listing of 610 drugs that had failed the government's own standards for effectiveness. All the drugs on Wolfe's list—which accounted for 169 million prescriptions, or one out of every 8 prescriptions filled in this country, and $1.1 billion in sales—were still being sold, and all had been available for at least eighteen and sometimes thirty years.

The government standards had been revised in 1962 as a result of federal legislation. Drugs issued before that time were retested by the National Academy of Sciences-National Research Council, under an FDA contract. DES was not in the book, because approval for its use during pregnancy had been withdrawn in 1971. But during its retesting stage it was found to be "possibly effective," a gracious description that meant that if controlled studies were done the results might or might not be negative. No drug company ever did those tests.

The drug industry has close ties with the medical profession, the group with the hands-on contact with consumers. In the early days of DES it was standard practice to list the name of the company providing the experimental drug in a footnote or other reference in a paper that was to be published. That practice has been largely dropped—for unknown reasons. It is therefore often impossible to read medical papers and know the sources of the drugs used.

The drug companies are very much aware of their vital financial interest in having doctors know about their products and prescribe them. Maura Sughrue, M.D., in Gainesville, Florida, kept track of every piece of free medical information she received during a one-month period from October 1 to November 1, 1981. The stack of material weighed twenty-three pounds and stood nine inches high, not including the parchmentlike scroll featuring Matthew Thornton, a signer of the Declaration of Independence. This last document, enclosed in a mailing tube and suitable for framing, was from Schering Corporation, which thoughtfully included a card offering free samples of Diprosone, a cream sold for inflammatory skin diseases.

The free journals Sughrue received during that month alone included issues of *Drug Therapy/Hospital; Infectious Diseases; Practical Cardiology; Family Practice News; Hospital Medicine; Hospital Practice; Private Practice; The Female Patient; Medical World News; The Journal of Family Practice; Family Practice Recertification; Patient Care;* and *Physician's Assets,* "a compendium of personal investment information."

She also received fliers advertising drugs from Smith Kline & French; McNeil Pharmaceutical; Roche Products; Merck Sharp & Dohme (whose flier included a 32-inch by 21-inch map of the world, with prescribing information for two of its products conveniently printed on the back); and an offer from a company for "a valuable gift worth up to $70!" for sending one or all of a series of illustrated medical texts to the medical or nursing student of her choice. The tests ranged in price from $24.50 (Vol. 1, *Nervous System*), to $47 (Vol. 7, *Respiratory System*) the complete set sold for $288, with a saving of $37 over the total cost of buying the volumes separately. The free gift for her included the choice of a Carry-on Duffle Bag by John Weitz, a Take-Along FM Stereo Mini Radio, a 32-ounce decanter, a quartz electronic alarm clock, or 7x35 prism binoculars.

During that one-month period she and other physicians in her group were treated to a free sandwich-and-potato-chip lunch by Roche Laboratories as a salesman pitched the benefits of its product Valium. Valium is a popular prescription tranquilizer that many health advocates contend is overprescribed with little regard for its potential addictive effect.

Here is one of the reasons drug companies like to stay on the good side of physicians, even if it's only through a free sandwich-and-potato-chip lunch. In March of 1982 Sughrue received a "Dear Doctor" letter from Roche Laboratories protesting what it called the "blatant misuse" of Valium in the movie *I'm Dancing as Fast as I Can*. The letter said the film "may generate serious, unjustified patient concerns and disrupt doctor/patient relationships . . . Nevertheless we believe that this film provides the public with a vivid example of what can occur when a medication is severely misused." In a hastily added P.S. a Roche official wrote that he had just learned of an upcoming segment of the Phil Donahue television show dealing with the same themes as the movie. The widely syndicated show "attacks Valium directly, the medical profession indirectly, and contains several references to the motion picture *I'm Dancing as Fast as I Can*. . . . The panel consists of two chemically dependent persons whose total problem is never clearly defined, combined with Jill Clayburgh (who stars in the film) and Sidney Wolfe, M.D., a purported consumer advocate."

Patricia McMillen, senior producer of *Donahue*, said, "It is not the intention of our television show to tell viewers what to do or what to think about a particular drug, but [in this case] to provide information about drug issues, and let women and men make up their own minds."

Wolfe was on the show to promote the most recent book from Public Citizen's Health Research Group, *Stopping Valium*, which describes what it calls health hazards to the more than 10 million Americans taking Valium and the estimated 8,000 people who are treated in hospital emergency rooms annually because of Valium addiction.

According to the Roche statement, "Dr. Wolfe, the only physician present, is asked, 'Is there ever a valid reason to prescribe Valium, in your opinion?' His answer, 'In my opinion, I would not prescribe it.' Such an inflammatory statement can only be viewed as a disservice to patients receiving therapy with Valium, and is likely to generate irrational fears."

The problem is, they left something out: while Wolfe had said he wouldn't prescribe Valium, he knew responsible physicians who would.

In view of the subtle pressure from drug companies hawking their wares, physicians have to be careful. Linda Johnston, M.D. (of Van Nuys, California), said drug company detail men "don't lie, but I'm more interested in what they don't say. I'm interested in medicine, and they're not. If I can get free samples that I know I want, it can be a benefit to the patient, saving them maybe twenty dollars on a prescription."

John Matrisciano, M.D., a Los Angeles surgeon, said: "A drug company salesman used to be the wise, older guy, similar to a hardware store guy—guys who knew how to do anything. Now the drug companies have hired chic, Madison Avenue-type women. Everybody gives me free samples."

New York hematologist-oncologist Neal Friedberg, M.D., told me: "There's no hard sell, and you can help patients with free samples. The drugs I use in my field are usually one-company drugs that have been developed for malignancies."

Dorothy Friedberg, M.D., an ophthalmologist, said: "I can be wary of drug company detail men. The medicines that are good you find out about through the literature. The detail men are walking advertisements for their companies—they're biased. In medicine you rely on the experience of people who have gone before you."

But some physicians have not always been careful. In 1978 former medical products salesman William MacKay, and journalist Maureen Mylander coauthored a book called *Salesman/Surgeon.* In this book he described how, in New York State, with no medical training, he had participated in numerous surgeries using equipment he sold. An investigation and several indictments against medical people (later dismissed), followed.

Caution should be the watchword whenever any drug is used, but especially during pregnancy. The contents of a pill or capsule can vary from manufacturer to manufacturer, and the impact of one ingredient can be modified by other ingredients. The human body is sensitive to everything. DES was made in a wide variety of compounds—some with vitamins, some without, by a wide variety of manufacturers in different parts of the country. The different pharmacologic properties of each make of drug differ; so will the impact. And the impact may vary depending upon whether a drug has been taken in the morning, the evening, on a full or empty stomach, and so on.

Look at aspirin. The June 24, 1981, issue of the *Medical Letter,* a nonprofit publication, took a look at aspirin products. It concluded: "Pharmaceutical differences between different brands of aspirin can have clinical consequences, but no controlled trials have been done to show that one brand of plain aspirin is a better analgesic than any other."

How much should patients know? How much should they be told? The FDA has been trying for some time to get complete package inserts included with every prescription drug sold. Package inserts list the chemical formula of the drug, the uses for which it is indicated, the situations in which it should not be used (contraindicated), and the potential side effects. In 1980 the drug industry's lobbying group, the Pharmaceutical Manufacturers Association, filed suit in federal court to stop the FDA from requiring a patient's package insert for birth control pills. (Birth control pills contain estrogen, which has been linked to endometrial cancer in women.) Joining the lawsuit against the FDA were the American College of Obstetricians and Gynecologists, the Congress of County Medical Societies, the Oklahoma State Medical Society, the American Society of Internal Medicine, the American Pharmaceutical Association, the National Association of Chain Drug Stores, and others. The FDA was supported by consumer groups, women's health organizations, and the Consumers Union of the United States.

The medical groups objected to the FDA ruling because it would, they claimed, interfere with the physician's ability to practice medicine. Concerns were voiced that patients might decide not to take the medicine after reading the insert, even though the medicine was vital for the patient's health, and therefore the physician should be allowed to determine whether or not a particular patient should receive the package insert. The FDA won in court, but full implementation of the order was halted by the Reagan Administration as part of its widespread efforts throughout the entire federal government to lessen the impact and power of federal watchdogs in order to deregulate American industries and "take the government off of people's backs."

That issue will doubtless come up again, perhaps in the case of another drug with the unrealized potency of DES; the $17 billion a year pharmaceutical industry has expressed concern in the past that the estimated ten years and $25 million it spends testing each new drug it brings out is too long a period of time and too great an expense for it to bear. If regulatory measures are loosened, as the Reagan administration wants, then the pharmaceutical companies might be able to bring new drugs out for less money in less time. That may make beneficial compounds available for health purposes; it may also bring new drugs on the market without full testing of their hazardous potentials.

The FDA lawsuit was one of the latest battles in the field of informed consent. Attorney William J. Curran pointed out in the December 24, 1981, issue of the *New England Journal of Medicine* that the complex issues involved "remain unanswered in today's rapidly changing world of improving, but still sometimes dangerous, prescription drug therapy."

What is the duty of the physician in warning the patient of either potential problems or newly discovered problems? None of the DES lawsuits has been against a physician. The accepted theory is that if a drug is approved for use by the FDA, the physician is following accepted medical practice in prescribing it. Liability rests with the drug manufacturer to test.

But that is changing.

In 1978 California's innovative appeals court ruled in *Tresemer* v. *Barke* that a physician has a duty to warn the patient of newly discovered problems, and that failure to do so can subject the physician to actions for negligence. The duty, in that case, existed because of a continuing relationship between the patient and the physician, who allegedly had not notified a woman of problems associated with the Dalkon shield intrauterine device. The device was inserted in 1972; by 1974 the problems were well known, and when it was removed in 1975, the patient had serious medical complications related to it. No money award was made in the case, but the principle stands. It has the potential to change the way medicine is practiced.

I went to interview a physician who is sympathetic to the DES consumer groups and skeptical of miracle drugs. We sat talking on the couch in his office when suddenly he got up in the middle of the conversation and put on his long white hospital coat. What was there about wearing that white hospital coat? Did he speak better wearing the coat? With more authority?

Doctors cure and heal and save lives. By virtue of that we have given them enormous power and authority over our bodies. Doctors belong to one of those few professions in democratic America in which a member is called by a title before his name. Unlike "Judge," and "Senator," and "Reverend" or "Rabbi," "Doctor So-and-So" puts his hands on our bodies, prescribes substances we ingest, helps us to get well. Perhaps this creates a bias in our minds, a tendency to embrace the title and trust the consequences. Surely physicians are among the best trained and best educated people in our society, but they too have their biases—*someone* is writing 169 million prescriptions annually for drugs that don't work.

But at the same time, there are people taking those pills. One physician, the retired head of a major university medical school, spoke eloquently about why DES didn't work, why the early tests were suspect, why he virtually never gave it. "But if a woman demanded it, then I wrote a prescription," he said. If a woman demanded it.

Doctors do want to help; that is their business, profession, intent, and calling. But no one wants to turn down a woman who, as one gynecologist remembers, "pounded her fist into her open hand and demanded I give her something. I refused, because I just don't like giving drugs during pregnancy, period. But others don't feel that way, and they are good doctors too. If we refuse to give a drug a woman demands, she'll find another doctor. That patient did."

Patients must take an active role in their own health care. The proliferation of popular books on a wide variety of medical topics and the availability in corner bookshops of the *Physicians' Desk Reference*, which contains information supplied by manufacturers on all drugs sold in the United States, attest to the growing awareness that consumers must inform themselves as fully as possible of medical complexities.

Medical care is what we make it. George Speck, M.D., remembers calming a DES mother about the chance of her daughter's getting cancer "while the daughter sat there, smoking cigarettes. I knew she was on the birth control pill. The risks associated with smoking and pill use are great and well known. Why was she smoking? Why was she taking the pill? Why wouldn't she listen to me when I told her about the risks?"

It can be dangerous for patients and physicians to assume that medical knowledge is ever complete on a given subject. Medical perceptions evolve over time as research continues to generate new findings or refine previous ideas. Even longtime DES foes were stunned when the cancer association in daughters was revealed. "It was like a bolt from the blue," said Michael B. Shimkin, M.D., who had showed its carcinogenic potential in animals. "It hit us in the face," said cancer authority Roy Hertz, M.D.

What if DES were synthesized today? To get on the market for use during pregnancy it would have to be shown to be safe and effective. With modern testing methods it could never be shown to be safe, and it has yet to be conclusively shown to be effective in preventing miscarriages. It might still be approved for use as an estrogen replacement in older women, a use for which it currently has FDA approval. But it might also exist as one of those compounds that enable scientists to study, in animals, how the body works. "DES may turn out to be a valuable molecule for demonstrating how a chemical substance can cause disturbances in different organs and functional systems, which are not immediately apparent, but interact in later malignant development," reported J.-G. Forsberg, of the University of Lund, Sweden, in a 1981 issue of the *International Journal of Biological Research in Pregnancy*. Used only in that way it might have achieved a prominence expected of it by Sir Edward Charles Dodds more than forty years ago, which was tainted instead by the problems that swirled around it—problems that are still being disentangled—when it was used during pregnancy.

From inventor to drug company to doctor to patient—the vital chain ties all aspects of the health community together. The forces of need, treatment, and marketing ebb and flow in an endless pattern, touching everyone involved. The chain begins somewhere, moves somehow, is influenced variously, but ends, always ends in the human body.

The woman is now in her thirties, has confirmed DES exposure, adenosis, and menstrual problems. She is married and has thought long and hard about the DES experience. She spoke of herself, for herself, but also for all the others.

"Its important in our relationship that we bring DES into focus and let those who are close to us know the greater depth of involvement that the DES experience has in our lives and theirs. DES now belongs to both of us, my husband and myself, because of the ongoing health question, the extra gynecological exams, and because of the question of children. It was hard for him at first—he had no place to put all this DES business, no way to make sense of it and understand it and digest it at the beginning. It was all new to him. And even though it wasn't new to me, it frightened me all over again because of everything that isn't known about the effects of DES exposure at this point in our lives. One night I was in bed reading about some new DES finding and I raised my voice, because he was shaving in the bathroom, to tell my husband about it. He came out and looked right at me and changed the subject. I started crying. I said 'What are you doing? I don't under-stand—I'm talking about something that's real important to me and you change the subject. What the hell are you doing?' He looked at me with a very wounded expression and said, 'I was only trying to take your mind off something I think you're stuck on in a very unhealthy way.' But I was scared, I needed support. Then he came to bed and just held me. He said, 'I'm sorry, I don't know as much as you do about DES and I'm not sure I really want to know.'"

Soft dark hair was touching her forehead with perspiration, from the heat of the evening, from the heat of the memory.

"I'm afraid of not being able to bear his children. I'm afraid of being a disappointment to him. I don't want someday to have to face that kind of 'failure'—that I'm inadequate because my 'equipment' doesn't function the way it should. And I don't have the emotional wherewithal to deal with that now.

"I put DES material in his briefcase when he was leaving for a trip. I told him that I'd put it there. Should I be offended if he didn't read it? I love him. If I allow myself to be resentful, I'm not doing either of us any good. What if we can't have children and the Ob-Gyn says, 'Here's this new medicine, this dandy new drug.' and I say, 'Show me all the studies that show it doesn't cause cancer or have harmful side effects on the fetus.' How will my husband react if he sees that drug as the only way for us to have children and I am saying, 'No, look at the possible consequences—it might be the DES story all over again'? How can he be expected to understand or accept that?

"I feel caught in a kind of schizophrenia. I'm active in advocating the right way of dealing with your body as a DES daughter, but when it comes to myself, I'm not so anxious to deal with it. I'm tired of trying to educate the doctors, because at heart they are Pollyannas—they believe in the good and the true and the beautiful, and they don't want to believe that this has taken place, under their noses, at their hands. . . ."

She paused. "Pain and suffering are the hardest things in the world to get at and to deal with. I feel as if I can't even trust myself on this issue, because deep down I've tried to keep my emotions bottled up. I've tried to be tough when it comes to DES, but, basically, I don't want to touch that spot of real insecurity. I'm very happy to be married, and I want to do the natural thing that most everybody does in their married lives— have children, a family. I have a lot of trouble balancing the informed picture I have of myself with the image we grow up with, heaven only knows where we get it—television, the movies, what have you—that all-American notion of the inalienable right to have a family that translates simply and naturally into having one. But it's not that simple. That image has been complicated and obscured. And now it involves anxiety—uncertainties about the future that have no hard-and-fast answers, and a real shaking up of the unquestioning, fundamental trust that you have always had in the medical world.

"How much of this should I discuss with my husband? How much of this doubt and anxiety should I try to deal with myself? It's not easy to have the presence of mind to ask all the questions that you want answers to when you're flat on your back on the doctor's examining table. Can I, should I, ask my husband to come to my exams and sit there and be an advocate for me, for us? I feel the need to have him there, to share this critical time of doubt and fear. There is a very deeply rooted and unfortunate attitude in our society, that female problems will always be just that: 'female problems.' Gynecology does not really live up to the meaning of its name, 'the study of woman.' At times it is treated more as an expected and forgivable ignorance.

"Is it possible people are better off not knowing about the ramifications of DES exposure? Sometimes it seems that way. But we have all got to come of age sooner or later, to be responsible to others, to enlighten the medical profession, to be responsible to and for ourselves. That's where we are now."

APPENDIX

1 - 800 - 225 - 6863

The following is a list of some of the organizations dealing with consumers and their health problems.

Coalition for the Medical Rights of Women
  1638-B Haight Street
  San Francisco, CA 94117
DES Action, National
  East Coast: Long Island Jewish Hospital, New Hyde Park, NY
    11040; (516) 775-3450
  West Coast: 1638-B Haight Street, San Francisco, CA 94117; (415)
    621-8032
Local:
  California: P.O. Box 205, 195 Claremont Avenue, Long Beach
              90803
              c/o YMCA, 1122 17 Street, Sacramento 95814
              1172 Morena Blvd., San Diego, 92110
              1638-B Haight Street, San Francisco 94117
              P.O. Box, 1185, Sunnymead 92110
  Connecticut: P.O. Box 70, Monroe 06468
  Florida: 9586 Portside Drive, Seminole 33542
  Hawaii: 95–710 Kipapa Drive #45, Milalani Town, 96789
  Illinois: P.O. Box 173, Park Forest 60466
  Louisiana: P.O. Box 6841, New Orleans 70174
  Massachusetts: P.O. Box 126, Stoughton 02072

Michigan: P.O. Box 2692, Ann Arbor 48106
2205 Rosewood SE, Grand Rapids 49506
Minnesota: 626 12th Avenue, Two Harbors, 55616
c/o YWCA, 1130 Nicollet Avenue, Minneapolis 55403
Missouri: c/o Cheryl Hermann, 4712 Milentz, St. Louis 63116
Montana: c/o Terri Tester, Rt. 1, P.O. Box 2950, Arlee 59821
Nevada: P.O. Box 5748, Reno 89513
New Hampshire: FRD #1, Epsom 03234
New Jersey: P.O. Box 323, Westwood 07675
P.O. Box 22, Fort Lee 07024
New Mexico: P.O. Box 40270, Albuquerque 87196
New York: Long Island Jewish Hospital, New Hyde Park 11040
North Carolina: Sherri Hopkins, 7512 Park Vista Circle, Pineville
28134
Ohio: Amy Edelman, 986 Quarry Drive, Cleveland 44121
P.O. Box 151113, Columbus 43215-0190
Oregon: P.O. Box 12092, Portland 97212
Pennsylvania: 340 Lenni Road, Glen Riddle 19037
Tennessee: 4101 McCahill Road, Chattanooga 37415
Texas: P.O. Box 1596, Spring 77373
Washington, D.C.: P.O. Box 5311, Rockville, MD 20851
Washington State: 2707 E. 18 Street, Spokane 99203
c/o Meschke, 2021 McElroy Place, Puyallup
98371
Wisconsin: 821 W. St. Francis, De Pere 54115
c/o Julie Pollak, 3729 N. Moris Blvd., Shorewood 53211
Canada: Snowdon, P.O. Box 233, Montreal, Quebec H3X 374

DES Registry, Inc., 5426 27 Street, N.W., Washington, D.C.
20015; (202) 966-1766
Public Citizen Health Research Group, 2000 P Street, N.W., #708,
Washington, D.C. 20036; (202) 872-0320
National Women's Health Network, 2025 "I" St., N.W. #105,
Washington, D.C. 20006; (202) 223-6886
RESOLVE (a consumer and information group dealing with infertil-
ity) P.O. Box 474, Belmont, Mass. 02178; (617) 484-2424

BIBLIOGRAPHY

The following is a list of some of the books mentioned in the text, as well as others of interest to consumers.

Bargmann, Eve, M.D., et al. *Stopping Valium and Ativan, Centrax, Dalmane, Librium, Paxipam, Restoril, Serax, Xanax.* Public Citizen's Health Research Group, 1982.

Bell, Susan E. *The Synthetic Compound Diethylstilbestrol (DES), 1938–1941.* Ph.D. dissertation, Brandeis University, 1980.

Bichler, Joyce. *DES Daughter.* Avon, 1981.

Epstein, Samuel S., M.D. *The Politics of Cancer.* Doubleday Anchor, 1979.

Fenichell, Stephen and Lawrence S. Charfoos. *Daughters at Risk: A Personal DES Story.* Doubleday, 1981.

Herbst, Arthur L., M.D. and Howard A. Bern, Ph.D. *Developmental Effects of Diethylstilbestrol (DES) in Pregnancy.* Thieme Stratton, Inc., 1981.

MacKay, William, and Maureen Mylander. *Salesman Surgeon.* McGraw-Hill, 1978.

Nilsson, Lennart. *Behold Man.* Little, Brown & Co., 1973.

Norwood, Christopher. *At Highest Risk: Protecting Children from En-*

vironmental Harm. McGraw-Hill, 1980; Penguin Books, 1981.

Orenberg, Cynthia Laitman. *DES: The Complete Story.* St. Martin's Press, 1981.

Sarath, Maria, et al. *Getting Yours: A Consumer's Guide to Obtaining Your Medical Records.* Public Citizen's Health Research Group, 1980.

Seaman, Barbara, and Gideon Seaman, M.D. *Women and the Crisis in Sex Hormones.* Bantam Books, 1977.

Wellford, Harrison. *Sowing the Wind. A Report from Ralph Nader's Center for Study of Responsive Law on Food Safety and the Chemical Harvest.* Grossman Publishers, 1972.

Wolfe, Sidney M., M.D., Christopher M. Coley, and the Public Citizen's Health Research Group. *Pills That Don't Work.* Farrar Straus & Giroux, 1980; Warner Books, 1982.

The following is a brief list of some of the medical articles mentioned most frequently in the text.

Ann B. Barnes, M.D., et al. "Fertility and Outcome of Pregnancy in Women Exposed *in Utero* to Diethylstilbestrol," *New England Journal of Medicine,* Vol. 302, No. 11, Mar. 13, 1980, pp. 609 ff.

Herbst, Arthur L., M.D., et al. "A Comparison of Pregnancy Experience in DES-Exposed and DES-Unexposed Daughters," *Journal of Reproductive Medicine,* Vol. 24, No. 2, Feb. 1980.

Herbst, Arthur L., M.D., et al. "Reproductive and Gynecologic Surgical Experience in Diethylstilbestrol-Exposed Daughters," *American Journal of Obstetrics and Gynecology,* Vol. 141, No., 1019, Dec. 15, 1981.

INDEX